Child Health Care in Āyurveda

Indian Medical Science Series No. 16

Child Health Care in Āyurveda

Dr. Abhimanyu Kumar
M.D. (Ay) Ph.D.

Sri Satguru Publications
A Division of
Indian Books Centre
Shakti Nagar, Delhi
INDIA

Published by :
Sri Satguru Publications
Indological and Oriental Publishers
A Division of
Indian Books Centre
40/5, Shakti Nagar,
Delhi-110007
(INDIA)

First Edition: Delhi, 1994

ISBN 81-7030-389-3

PRINTED IN INDIA
Mehra Offset Press
Darya Ganj, Delhi

Contents

Contents

Preface

> "Disease is very old, and nothing about it has changed. It is we who changed, as we learn to recognise what was formerly impereceptible."
>
> **-Jean Martin Charcot**

The history of medicine is at the same time a very old and a very young field of study. It is not a mear history concerned of only historians, but is equally important for medical professionals too. Medical history tells us where we came from and where we stand in art of healing at present. Several generations of philologists and historians have made source available to us. Truely speaking, medical history is the compass that guides us into the future and shows the direction in which we are marching.

History of medicine practiced by Indians is much interesting than the medical system of any other country. In 1920, Indian archaeologists discovered large cities in the Indus Valley. The chief sites excavated so far are Mohanjodaro and Harappa. Culture of these cities much have florished in the 3000 B.C. It would be matter of great curiosity that what kind of medicine was practiced those days by Indus people. No any kind of text or document we find related to that. It can be merely an idea that medicine practiced those days must have been similar to that of other peoples of similar period, like of Sumer and Creta. The medicine may be a combination of religions, magical and empirical rites and procedures.

Vedas are the source of all science and learning of Indians, after the Aryan invasion, Ancient scholars received knowledge from their ancestors and compiled in the form of four *Vedas* - *Ṛgveda, Yajurveda, Sāmveda* and *Atharvaveda.* These are consisted of hymns, prayers, incantations and ritual formulas. Commentaries of *Veda* were written later on as *Brāhmaṇas, Āraṇyakas* and *Upaniṣadas. Ṛgveda* and particularly *Atharvaveda* were concerned with matter of health care. *Vedic* medicine must have flourished for centuries and Indian medicine, thereafter was named, *Āyurveda.*

Āyurveda is a science that imparts the knowledge concerned to life, the main aim being to provide guidelines for maintenance and promotion of health, as well as prevention and treatment of diseases. In other words, *Āyurveda* is a science which helps in understanding creative and non-creative aspects of life, happy and un-happy life; congenials and ṇon-congenials for life; life span and also corporal dimensions. It consists of eight clinical branches, namely - *Kāyacikitsā* (General medicine), *Śalya* (Surgery), *Śālākya* (Eye and E.N.T.), *Agada Tantra* (Toxicology), *Bhūta Vidya* (study related to intervention of supernatural powers), *Kaumārabhṛtya* (Child health care), *Rasāyana* (Rejuvenative, anabolic and preventive methods), *Vājīkaraṇa* (methods for achieving energy and sexual power).

Kaumārabhṛtya (child health care) has been considered as an important speciality of *Āyurveda.* Various terms have been used for this, during ancient period, viz. *Kaumārabhṛtyakam, Kaumārabhṛtya, Kaumāratantra, Bālacikitsā, Darakatikicchā* or *Bāla Roga.*

The word *'Kaumārabhṛtya'* is composed of two words - *Kumāra* and *Bhṛtya.* The word *'Kumāra'* was used in *Vedas,* in the sense of a child, boy, youth, son, etc., while in Saṃskṛt literature this word has been specially used for Kārtikeya, the son of Lord Śivā. The children of royal families were also called *Kumāra*.

The word *'Kumāra'*, being pole of the subject needs further analysis, which is combination of two words - *Ku* and *māra*. According to the lexicon of M.M. William, the word *'Ku'* is used as a prefix implying deterioration, depreciation or deficiency. The word *'māra'* is derived from root *'mṛī'* means easily dying; while in Saṁskṛt literature the word *'mār'* is used as a synonym of the God of love (*Kāmadeva*). In the present context, i.e., in strict medical sense *'Kāmadeva'* can be correlated with the sex hormones. As described in Saṃskṛt literature, *Kāmadeva* is mainly responsible for sexual activities, including the physical constitution of body. In the same way sex hormones are also responsible for development of sex organs, constitution of body and lastly for sexual activities. It is well accepted fact as per modern medical sciences, that sex organs are not fully developed mature in the childhood period.

The discussion clearly shows that childhood is the period during which sex hormones (*Kāmadeva*) are deficient (*ku*) and sex organs are not fully mature. Keeping in view these facts, our ancient scholars decided to limit this stage of life (childhood) upto fifteen/sixteen years. Generally a person becomes sexually mature, after this period. These thoughts of ancient scholars resemble with those of the scientists of modern era. *'Bhṛtya'* word is originally, derived from root *'bhrne bharaṇe'* means to bear (in womb), wear, nourish, support and maintain. *Raghuvaṃśa* of Kālidāsa also supports the meaning of this word, as this is used for care of young child or for care of a woman in pregnancy.

Above description clearly shows that the word *'Kaumārabhṛtya'* is coined for the subject, which is mainly concerned with the maintenance along with the care of child. Experts of this speciality are known as '*Kaumārabhṛtya Bhiṣak*' and their nature of work has been considered very tough than experts of other specialities of *Āyurveda.*

Various scholars of ancient period have described the field of *Kaumārabhṛtya* in their own way but the broader area covered is more or less the same. Before the period of *Caraka,* no one has described the field of *Kaumārabhṛtya* clearly. However, *Caraka* also referred only the name of the subject but not explained the scope of the subject. *Cakrapāṇi,* the commentator of *Caraka Saṃhitā,* has defined the subject and said that *bharaṇa* of *Kumāra* is the main area of *Kaumārabhṛtya.*

Suśruta has very vividly explained the subject matter of *Kaumārabhṛtya.* It includes:

(i) Nursing and healthy upbringing of infants and children.

(ii) Purifying and improvement of breast milk found deficient in quality and quantity.

(iii) Treatment of:

  a. diseases due to the use of vitiated breasted milk.
  b. diseases peculiar found in infant and childhood period.
  c. diseases due to influence of *grahas.*

Suśruta has further elaborated the subject. The features of all the nine *grahas,* treatment of *Skanda,* etc. *bāla grahas,* gynaecological disorders and the subject described in *Śārīra Sthāna* of *Suśruta Samhitā,* are included in *Kaumārabhṛtya. Dalhaṇa,* commenting on the verse says that physiology of menstruation and descend of embryo, etc. are described in *Śārīra sthāna* of *Suśruta Saṃhitā* also come under the perview of *Kaumārabhṛtya.*

Childhood is a very tender but superb stage of human life. The effect of physical development and mental status of this stage have its effect over rest of the life period. During this stage the *dhātus* are immature: therefore, special care of this stage is very essential. Almost all the scholars have considered the upper limit of this stage upto 16 years. *Vāgbhaṭa,* at one place, has considered this upto 10 years.

On the basis of references available childhood period may be further sub-divided into 3 stages-*Kṣīrapa, Kṣīrānnāda,* and *Annāda. Kaśyapa* has somewhat different opinion from other scholars and described 3 stages - *garbha, bāla* and *kumāra.* By the description, it can be inferred that except *Kaśyapa* all other have given the classification on the basis of feeding pattern of child, while *Kaśyapa's* classification is based on physical developmental states.

Suśruta has determined three stages of childhood as *Kṣīrāda* (from birth upto one year of age), *Kṣīrānnāda* (1-2 year), *Annāda* (above 2 year age).

Kaśyapa has little difference of opinion. He has included *Kṣīrānnāda* stage in *Annāda,* and termed *Bāla* to *Kṣīrapa* and *Kumāra* to the *Annāda. Kṣīrapa* (*bāla*) from birth to one year and *Annada* (*kumāra*) from 1 year to 16 years.

The upper age limit of female child has been also considered upto sixteen years. *Hārita* has further classified this period and considered that upto 5 years the girl is *Bālā,* upto eleven years *Mugdhā* or by other classification *Bāla* upto twelve years, and *Mugdhā* upto the age of 19 years. This difference may be considered as individual variation. *Pārāśara Smṛti* has categorised childhood period of female child into four stages - *Gaurī* (upto 8 years), *Rohiṇī* (upto 9 years), *Kanyā* (upto 10 years), and *Rajomatī* after this stage.

The references of the subject, found scattered in ancient literature have been recapitulated and discussed in the book under different Chapters. The Chapter 'Care of newborn' deals with various aspects related to newborn like resuscitation, feeding, protective measures and general care. These are the original contributions of *Āyurvedic* scholars like *Caraka* and *Suśruta,* though the concepts are also available in Buddhist and Jain literature. The concept 'Breast is best' really come from *Vedic* period. Role of *dhātrī* (wet-nurse) has been considered very vital and discussed in chapter on Infant feeding. The Chapter 'General Care of Children' covers protective measures, proper handling and psychological Care of Child. Unique description available in ancient texts regarding dentition, has been mentioned in a separate Chapter. *Saṃskāras* are considered the main field of *Gṛhya Sūtras,* though the concepts are also available in *Āyurvedic* texts.

Ancient *Āyurvedic* scholars have kept the provision of clinical examination of healthy child for assessing his longevity and a diseased for diagnosis of disease. The description is included in Chapter 'Clinical examination of Children'. Ample references are available regarding principles of treatment and drug therapy of Children. Initially the texts of ancient period have discussed only about the specific problems of children, but in the literature of later period, recipes for some common diseases, especially formulated for children have been described, are discussed in a separate Chapter 'Diseases of Children and their treatment.'

In brief, the science of child health care was cultivated from very ancient time in India. Even in *Vedic* literature, there are reference to Children's diseases. Religious texts like *Gṛhya sūtras* and *smṛtis,* etc. are mainly concerned with the description of *Saṃskāras. Garbhopaniṣada* deals exclusively with fetal development. Prediction of Congenital Malformations could be done on the basis of the concepts described in *Bṛhata Jātaka.* Buddhist and Jain literature have references of feeding of newborn, concepts of *dhātrī* and about very few diseases. *Saṃskṛta* literature mostly deals with the care of newborn. *Āyurvedic* texts have included all the aspects of child health care. *Kaśyapa* has given supreme importance to the speciality of child health care.

Review of all available texts gives a picture that the scholars, after *Agniveśa* (*Caraka Saṃhitā*), have started adding the description of diseases specific to the children. This trend has advanced with the time and scholars of later period have included mostly the recipes for treatment providing easy and quick formularies to the physicians. The references clearly indicate that this branch was fully developed in ancient period and the contributions are still highly relevant and up-to-date.

Acknowledgements - I pay my humble respect with deep sense of gratitude to Prof. C. Chaturvedi, B.H.U. Varanasi, who gave me scientific searchlight at every stage and has been kind enough to extend his able guidance in each and every step in completing the present work. Prof. (Km.) P.V. Tewari, Head of the department of *Prasūti Tantra* and Dean Faculty of *Āyurveda,* Institute of Medical Sciences, B.H.U. Varanasi gave me constant encouragement, suggestions and maternal affection throughout the present work and accepted my request to write the Introduction of the book. Gratuitous praise and immense gratitude are the least that I can offer to her. I have a profound sense of gratitude to Dr. R.D. Sharma Reader, Department of *Prasūti Tantra,* IMS, B.H.U. for his constant encouragement.

With great reverance and gratitude I humbly offer regards at the feet of my worshipable and beloved father Shri N.R. Dhangar, Asstt. Commissioner and mother Smt. Vindeshwari Devi whose constant love and blessing, inspiration and aspiration reflected me in the present position. I find no appropriate words to express my feelings to my wife (Mrs.) Shakuntala for her even encouraging and supporting attitude during the entire period of the work. Very special thanks are due to my sweet daughters Aditi and Ankita to keep me relaxed with their innocent smiles, during this stearnuous job.

Last but not the least I extend my thanks to M/s. Indian Books Centre for presenting this book before you expeditiously in such a elegant manner.

19th Nov. 1993 **Abhimanyu Kumar**

Introduction

Āyurveda, the science of life, considered as *Upaveda or Upāṅga* of *Rigveda* or *Atharvaveda,* in fact originated prior to *Vedas,* because the flora or plant kingdom, the basis source material for treatment came into existence earlier to the mankind, and the human being knew the method to protect, nurture and procreate ownself by intrinsic or inherent knowledge, much before he knew to express or scribe, that is why the *Āyurveda* is said to be preached by god of creation i.e. *Brahmā,* who created gods, demons, ancestors, human-being, seven domeṣtic and wild animals alongwith drugs (herbal drugs) and plant kingdom simultaneously.[1]

When *Vedas* were being written, subject of *Āyurveda* was also included, with relatively more quantum found in *Atharvaveda.* Due to this fact *Kaśyapa* though showing faith in *Atharvaveda* considers *Āyurveda* as fifth *Veda,* rather more important, strong and dominant, as *Āyurveda* is equated with thumb while other four *Vedas* with four fingers of palm.[2] Because of its eternity, it is said to have descended from heaven to earth, which passage was facilitated by the sages having gone to *Indra* to learn it.

1. *Kā. S. Kalpa. Revatī Ka.*/3.
2. *Kā. S. Vimā. Śiṣ.*/10.

Āyurveda though present in *Vedas* in abundance, but is not in a systemetised way. With the advancement of knowledge, thus, in the process of systemetization first stage is description of three principles (*trisūtra*) or three pillars[1] (*triskandha*) denoting basic tenets for diagnosis and treatment, while for practical applicability with specialization, it is divided in eight branches amongst which *Kaumārabhṛtya* is one, which is considered to be first or foremost in *Kāśyapa saṃhitā,*[2] the only source book of the subject available today.

Normal healthy *Strī-bīja* (ovum) and *Puṃbīja* (sperm) of the parteners possessing pure psyche, propelled by normal *Vāyu,* travelling through well functioning genital tract of respective partner unite inside the *Kukṣi* (uterus-fallopian tubes), wherein *Jīva* also descend.[3] This *garbha* after being nourished then delivered at appropriate time by the mother is further nurtured by her own breast-milk and then after proper growth and development, become a *Kumāra.* Naturally to obtain physically and psychologically healthy *Kumāra,* it is imperative for the physician to know above described entire process, which is the subject of obstetrics and gynaecology. This *Kaumārabhṛtya* actually encompasses two specialities of today i.e. obstetrics with gynaecology and paediatrics with neonatology. Now the knowledge has advanced considerably, thus, has necessitated that *Āyurveda* be now divided in more branches, Professor P.V. Sharma has advanced the idea of sixteen division of *Āyurveda* in his book[4] in which *Prasūtītantra* with *Strī roga* and *Kaumārabhṛtya* are given the status of independent specialities. In practice *Prasūtītantra* and *Strī roga* (obstetrics and gynaecology) and

---

1. *C. S. Sū. 1/24, 25.*
2. *C.S. Sū. 30/20, 28; S.S. Sū. 1/6, 7; A.S. Sū. 1/10; A.H. Sū. 1/5* and *Kā. S. Vi. Śiṣ. /10.*
3. *C.S. Śā. 8/17; S.S. Śā. 2/33; A.S. Śā. 1/68* and *A.H. Śā. 1/8, 9.*
4. *"Ṣoḍaśāṅga Hṛdayaṃ".* Pub. by Padmā Prakāśana 1987.

bāla-roga (paediatrics with neonatology) are now taught and examined separately at graduate and post graduate level in all the *Āyurvedic* institutions, however, the department is still one. The National Institute of Āyurveda, Jaipur has taken a lead in correct direction and has established separate departments of *Kaumārabhṛtya* and *Prasūtitantra* with *Strī roga.* This is high time that all other institutions also follow the suit.

To procure, protect and caress once own progeny is a basic instinct of every living being, naturally the subject related to this *Kaumārabhṛtya* finds relatively important place in ancient literature.

Vedas the first written record of India contain large number of references pertaining to this subject. To get a child of high intellect, the prayers were offered during fetal stage,[1] in other words the basic idea that mental faculties have good growth during intra-uterine life was accepted. Mother (*Aditi*) gave *soma-rasa* to *Indra* before feeding her own breast.[2] This form is practised even to day as first feed of glucose water is given to newborn followed by milk. To get a son possessing virility and prowess prayers were offered to various gods,[3] concept of wet-nurse was also existing.[4]

For protection of just delivered child the fire was prayed,[5] probably due to its high bactericidal and cleansing power. Specific hymn to be recited before feeding ceremony was mentioned.[6] Detailed management of a child is given in which *Vrīhi* etc. drugs were used for protection of child, it

1. *R.V.I. 119-7.*
2. *R.V. III. 48-2.*
3. *R.V.I. 98-7; III. 36-10; III-53-1* and *18; IV-1-3; IV-2-5, 11* and *18 etc.*
4. *R.V.I. 95-1* and 2.
5. *A.V. XX. 96-13.*
6. *A.V. VIII. 2-1* with comm. by *Sāyaṇācārya.*

was indicated that cloths covering the child should be pleasurable; tonsure, *Godāna* and *Upanayana* (threading ceremany) *Saṃskāras* were performed, it was accepted that cereals are basic substance to increase strength, if used improperly can cause loss of strength; the child initially swallows/digests cereals with difficulty, but afterwards eats easily *ie.* a milestone of growth and development of digestive capacity as well as requirements of the body; the drugs growing round the year provide health and pleasure.[1]

The fire, *Mitrāvaruṇa* and *Aditi* were prayed to bestow the child with all the qualities, make him free from diseases, protect him from *Piśāca* etc. demons so that he attains old age or lives upto old age;[2] for attainment of old age with disease - free state *Indra* etc. gods were also prayed.[3]

It was accepted that disease *Kāsa* (cough) influences each and every part of body, for its eradication the sun is prayed and living in hills or forest was advised,[4] similarly for *Yakṣmā* nourising oblation (*havi*), heat of sun, fresh air, heat of fire etc. were advised.[5] It appears that *Kāsa* and *Yakṣmā* refer to tuberculosis, for which above mentioned treatment is accepted even today as most important. Sun is prayed for eradication of other diseases also,[6] which indicates that bactericidal properties of sun-rays were recognised.

Disease *Grāhi* probably *Graha-rogas* of *Āyurvdic* classics seizes the child,[7] *Daśavṛkṣa* is prayed for it treatment,[8]

---

1. *A.V. VIII. 2-14* to *22* with comm. by *Sāyaṇācārya.*
2. *A.V. II. 28* complete with comm. by *Sāyaṇācārya.*
3. *A.V. III. 11* complete.
4. *A.V.I. 12-3* and *III-11-1* with comm. by *Sāyaṇācārya.*
5. *A.V. III. 1* complete with comm. by *Sāyaṇācārya.*
6. *A.V. I-12-1* to *4.*
7. *R.V.X. 103* complete and 161-1; *Yaju XVII. 44.*
8. *A.V. II. 9* complete.

besides prayers to other dieties are also offered,[1] *Yātudhānī* also similar to *Bālagraha* of *Āyurvedic* classics produces unconsciousness and attempts to suck *Rasa* or blood of the child.[2] The breasts enchanted with hymn were advised to be offered to the child seized with *Jambhā*,[3] or the milk poured over *Priyaṅgu* and rice pieces was advised to be given to the child.[4]

The disease transmitted to the children by parents suffering from *Kṣaya, Kuṣṭha,* etc. was termed as *Kṣetriya,* and for its eradication prayers,[5] *Śṛṅga* (horn), drugs and medicated water were used.[6] Similar large number of reference of the subject are found in *Vedas,* the author has referred those at appropriate places.

As *Kaumārabhṛtya* deals with the subject related to procurement of once own progeny, a highly cherished desire of human being, maximum *Saṃskāras* and religious worships i.e. *Garbhādhāna, Puṃsawana, Sīmantonnayana, Kṣipraprasawana, Jātakarma, Upaveśana, Annaprāśana, Chūḍākaraṇa, Karṇavedhana* and *Upanayana* etc. are performed during this stage; the features of pregnant woman i.e. *Dauhṛda* denote physical and psychological character of the child, thus, has attracted the attention of writers of all ages, naturally abundant material is found not only in *Vedas* but *Upaniṣad, Smṛties, Purāṇas, Gṛhyasūtras* and other *Saṃskṛta* epics alongwith Bauddha and Jain literature. The author has fathomed this vast sea to pick up beeds scattered here and there and has chained them appropriately so that a good beautiful garland of subject has emerged.

---

1. *A.V. VI. 112-1, 2* and *VI-113-1* and *3.*
2. *A.V.I. 28-3* and *4; IV-17-3.*
3. *A.V. VII. 10.*
4. *Kau. Sū.* XXXII-1-2.
5. *A.V. II. 8* and *10* complete with comm. by *Sāyaṇācārya.*
6. *A.V. III. 7* - complete.

Amongst various Āyurvedic classics available today only one book i.e. *Kāśyapa saṃhitā* is a book of this speciality, of which hardly one fourth part of its original contents is available today, which is not sufficient to impart knowledge sufficient to any specialist of the subject. Other classics though belong mainly to two branches i.e. *Kāyacikitsā* and *Śalya* alongwith *Śālākya* but provide sufficient scope for inter-disciplinary knowledge, albeit the relevant material is spreaded over entire classics, naturally one has to dive deep in order to collect the subject matter of one's speciality and then has to arrange them in such a systemic order, that the reader acquires sufficient knowledge. The author has done this commendable job, and described the subject under specific chapters.

Knowledge of any subject more so-over of science is never static, new theories and ideas replace the older one, though it is not so with *Āyurveda,* the hypothesis expounded by sages thousands of years back are true and applicable even today, but due to scarce availability of writing material during those ancient dyas, only principles are scribed and the details which were transmitted through direct preachings are lost in oblivion, due to discontinuity of traditions, as a result of foreign invasion. To understand these principles correctly it is imperative to take help of available literature of other systems of medicine, namely Allopathic or modern medicine. Due to drastic change in socio-cultural, economic and environmental status, new diseases and challanges have also cropped up, which cannot be over looked or discarded and had to be incorported within overall frame of *Āyurveda.* Author has very correctly and tactfully used this knowledge of modern medicine to explain *Āyurveda* as well as to make the book complete, so that the reader becomes equipped with sufficient knowledge and is able to practice with good command.

Today the trend has changed and the attitude of hatred towards ancient and old has transformed into longings, thus, the westerners are getting more and more interested in ancient culture, traditions and medicine of India. However, the languge of traditional classics comes as a big barrier for majority of them. The English language used by the author has overcome this hurdle and will be an instrument for dissemination of knowledge to a much wider population of globe.

The chapterization of subject and method of presentation is highly intelligible.

By writting the book in English, incorporating the subject matter available in wide spectrum of literature as well as almost all available *Āyurvedic* classics of ancient period, the author has bridged the gap being felt by majority of inquisitive and enthusiastic students of *Āyurveda.*

I am sure that the pace of this young intelligent, deligent writer of great potentials will not slow down and he will continue to worship the goddess *Sarasvatī* in all future days to come and serve the *Āyurveda.*

Prof. (Kum.) P.V. Tewari
Dean & Head
Faculty of Ayurveda
Department of Prasuti Tantra
Institute of Medical Sciences,
Banaras Hindu University,
Varanasi - 221 005

Abbreviations

Ācārādhyāya	Ācā
Āpastamba Gṛhya Sūtra	Āp. Gṛ. Sū.
Āpastamba Dharma Sūtra	Āpas. Dha.
Atharva veda	A.V.
Aśauca prakaraṇa	Aśau.
Āśvalāyana Gṛhya Sūtra	Āśwa. Gṛ. Sū.
Aṣṭānga Saṃgraha	A.S.
Aṣṭānga Hṛdaya	A.H.
Aitareya Brāhmaṇa	Ait. B.
Brhajjābāla Upaniṣada	Brhajjā. U.
Brhadāraṇyaka Upaniṣada	Brhadā U.
Baudhāyana Dharma Sūtra	Baudhā Dha.
Brahmacārī Prakaraṇa	Brahm
Caraka Saṃhitā	C.S.
Cikitsā Kalikā	C.K.
Chāndogya Upaniṣad	Chāndo. U.
Dvitīya Sthāna	Dwi. Sthā.
Garbhopaniṣada	Garbho. U. or G.U.
Gobhila Gṛhya Sūtra	Go. Gṛ. Sū.
Gautama Dharma Sūtra	Gaut. Dha.

Garuṇa Purāṇa	Garuṇa Pu.
Hārīta Saṃhitā	Hā.S.
Harmekhalā	H.M.
Hiraṇyākeśīya Gṛhya Sūtra	Hi. Gṛ. Su.
Jātisūtrīya Adhyāya	Jāti
Kalyāṇa Kāraka	K.K.
Kalpa Sthāna	Ka.
Kāśyapa Saṃhitā	K.S.
Kaṭha Upanisad	Kaṭh. U.
Kāṭhaka Gṛhya Sūtra	Kā. Gṛ. Su.
Kaivalya Upaniṣad	Kaival. U.
Kauśītakī Upaniṣad	Kauśī. U.
Khadira Gṛhya Sūtra	Kha. Gṛ. Su.
Manu Smṛti	Manu. Smṛ.
Māṇḍūkya Upaniṣad	Māṇḍū. U.
Mādhava Nidāna	M.N.
Nāvanitakam	Nāv
Nidāna Sthāna	Ni.
Nārāyaṇa Upaniṣad	Nārāy. U.
Prathama Sthāna	Pra. Sthā.
Pañcama Sthāna	Pañ. Sthā.
Pāraskara Gṛhya Sūtra	Pā. Gṛ. Sū.
Pārāśara Smṛti	Pārā. Smṛ.
Praśna Upaniṣad	Praś. U.
Prāyascittādhyāya	Prāy.
Ṛgveda	R.V.
Suśruta Saṃhitā	S.S.
Sūtra Sthāna	Sū.
Śārīra Sthāna	Śā.

Siddhi Sthāna	Si.
Saṣṭha Sthāna	Sas. Stha.
Śatapatha Brāhmaṇa	Śat. B.
Śāṃkhāyana Gṛhya Sūtra	Śā. Gṛ. Su.
Sāmvidhāna Brāhmaṇa	Sām. B.
Sāmveda	S.V.
Sāhasa Prakaraṇa	Sāha.
Tṛtīya Sthāna	Tṛ. Sthā.
Uttara Tantra	U.
Vaśiṣṭha Dharma Sūtra	Vaśi. Dha.
Vivāha Prakaraṇa	Vivā.
Viṣṇu Dharma Sūtra	Vis. Dha.
Viṣṇu Smṛti	Viṣṇu Smṛ.
Vrahata Jātaka	V.J.
Vaikhānasa Smārta Sūtra	Vaikhā. Sma.
Vyavahārādhyāya	Vya.
Vṛnda Vaidyaka	V.V.
Yajurveda	Y.V.
Yatidharma Prakaraṇa	Yati.
Yājñyavalka Smṛti	Ya. Smṛ.
Yama Smṛti	Yama. Smṛ.

Key to Transliteration

अ	a	घ	gha	प	pa
आ	ā	ङ	ṅa	फ	pha
इ	i	च	ca	ब	ba
ई	ī	छ	cha	भ	bha
उ	u	ज	ja	म	ma
ऊ	ū	झ	jha	य	ya
ऋ	ṛ	ञ	ña	र	ra
ॠ	r	ट	ṭa	ल	la
ए	e	ठ	ṭha	व	va
ऐ	ai	ड	ḍa	श	śa
ओ	o	ढ	ḍha	ष	ṣa
औ	au	ण	ṇa	स	sa
अं	ṃ	त	ta	ह	ha
अ:	Ḥ	थ	tha	क्ष	kṣa
क	ka	द	da	त्र	tra
ख	kha	ध	dha	ज्ञ	jña
ग	ga	न	na		

1

Care of Newborn

Normally, the fetus is mature upto 9th-10th month and gets ready to come out of the womb.[1] Delivery is a complicated process and also has its effect on fetus. Prayers for safe delivery have been offered in Atharva Veda. 'At this birth, O Pushan, let Aryaman (as) efficient invaker utter vāṣaṭ for thee, let the woman, rightly engendered, be relaxed let her joints go apart in order to birth'.[2]

'Four are the directions of the sky, four also of the earth; the gods sent together the fetus; let them unclose her in order to birth'.[3]

'Let Pushan (?) unclose (her or it); we make the yoni go apart, do thow, Sūṣaṇā, loosen; do thou biṣkalā, let go'.[4]

Now, as it were stuck (āhata) is the flesh, not in the fat, not as it were in the marrow, let the spotted slimy (?) after birth came down, for the dog to eat; let the after birth descend'.[5]

'I split apart thy urinator, apart the yoni, apart the (two) groin, apart both the mother and the child, apart the boy from the after birth; let the after birth descend'.[6]

'As the wind, as the mind, as fly the birds so do thou, O ten month's (child), fly along with the after birth; let the after birth descend'.[7]

First born of the after birth, the ruddy (Usriya) bull, born of wind and cloud (?), goes thundering with rain; may he be the merciful to our body, going straight on, breaking; he who, one force, hath stridden out three-fold'.[8]

The time, at which the child is delivered, may also has it's bad effect on his parents. Description is available in Atharva Veda to alay such type of effects. If the child is delivered in Jyeṣṭhā Nakṣatra, the birth of the child may be fatal for his brother, parents and other family members. For protection from the effect of Jyeṣṭhā Nakṣatra, Lord Agni has been prayed.[9] In Buddhist literature, the term 'Jātaka' has been used for newborn.[10]

The description related to care of newborn can be divided into following broad headings and sub-headings:

1. Immediate Care of Newborn
   - (a) Resuscitation of normal baby
   - (b) Resuscitation of unconscious or asphyxiated baby
   - (c) Cutting of umbilical cord
2. General Care
   - (a) Bath
   - (b) Feeding
   - (c) Bed and Cloths, and
   - (d) Protective measures.

1. Immediate Care of Newborn (Prāṇapratyāgamana)

Care of newborn, immediately after delivery, is vital step because any mis-management at this stage may prove fatal to the baby. The description of the subject matter available in various ancient texts is systematically arranged as follows:

(a) *Resuscitation of normal baby*

The literature before Caraka[11] had not mentioned any specific description regarding resuscitation of normal newborn. Caraka has prescribed following steps to resuscitate a normal newborn.

1. Sound should be produced by stricking or rubbing two stones together, near the base of the ear of newborn.
2. Hot or cold water should be sprinkled over face of the child. Cakrapāṇi has clarified that hot water is used in summer while cold in winter, for this purpose.

By these two processes, normally, the child gets relief from the trouble caused during the process of delivery and it regain the life. After proper resuscitation, the orifices are cleaned and bath is given.

3. For proper cleaning of oral cavity (including palate, lips, throat and tongue), the attending pediatrician should use his properly cleaned finger, whose nail has already been trimmed. Finger end must be wrapped with cotton.
4. Once the child is properly cleaned, the brahma-randhra (ant. fontanelle) should be protected by putting a cotton pad, soaked in oil (Balā Taila).
5. For removal of swallowed garbhodaka (liquor amnii), emesis should be induced by administering ghṛta mixed with saindhava (rock salt), to the new born.
6. Cutting of umbilical cord and Jātakarma should be performed according to the rituals.

After completing these processes, the first feed of madhu and ghṛta is offered.

Suśruta[12] has changed the sequence of processes for resuscitation but had described most the processes similar to Caraka and omitted the process of stimulation of newborn by a sound produced with the help of two stones.

1. Just after birth, ulva (vernix caseosa) should be removed from the body and oral cavity is to be cleaned by using saindhava lavaṇa (rock salt) and ghṛta.

2. Mūrdhā (ant. fontanellae) is to be cared of by covering it with tampoon soaked in ghṛta or Balā-taila, followed by cutting of umbilical cord.
3. If the child is unconscious due to compression of yoni and/or by instruments (asphyxiated) should be revived by sprinkling cold water.
4. Jātakarma is performed by licking the mixture of honey, ghṛta and powder of anantā (gold) in the dose of one guñjā, by index finger.
5. Bath should be given after massaging with Balā-taila.

Vāgbhaṭa[13] has mentioned that after cleaning the ulva (vernix caseosa), the revival of deeply unconscious baby should be done by pouring Balā-taila on head and making sound by stricking of two stones (details under resuscitation of unconscious newborn). Cutting of umbilical cord, bath, protection of tālu, cleaning of oral cavity and emesis for removal of swolled garbhodaka have been advised as described by Caraka and Suśruta.

Aṣṭānga Hṛdaya[14] has similar description to that of Aṣṭānga Saṃgraha for resuscitation of newborn. Other texts like Kalyāṇa Kāraka,[15] Cakradatta[16] and Yogaratnasamuccaya[17] have followed previous authors. However, Cakradatta[18] has mentioned a separate recipe for inducing emesis to remove Garbhodaka. For this purpose powder of Śuṇṭhī, Kṛṣna marica, Pippalī, Harītakī, Vacā and Haridrā mixed in breast milk should be given to newborn.

(b) *Resuscitation of unconscious/asphyxiated newborn*

Usually, most of the newborns revive without any special effort, however, few may suffer from deep unconsciousness (birth anoxia).

Mārkaṇḍeya Purāṇa is of the opinion that after delivery the newborn may be deeply unconcious but he attain consciousness after contact with atmosphere.[19]

Notable text of Āyurveda, Caraka Saṃhitā mentioned, if, the child does not respond with above mentioned methods, then fanning with winnowing basket made of Kṛṣṇakapālikā (isikā or nala muñja - vaṃśa) or a blackened broken earthen pot,[20] should be done till the child fully revives.

Vāgbhaṭa is of opinion that if, the child is suffering from fever, deep unconsciousness, does not cry, or his dhātus are decreased or unstable, and has too much pain on touching and the child looks like almost dead; he should be irrigated with Balā-taila and fanning with Winnowing basket (blackened by applying smoke),[21] should be done. Mantra should be enchanted in the right ear of newborn.[22]

"Thou is born from different body parts and from the heart. Ātmā itself is named as son. Thou live for hundred years, in which each years should be hundred years. Thou attain longevity nakṣatras (planets), diśās (directions), nights and days should protect thy."

Such child, if not revived properly may have various serious complications (cerebral palsy, etc.) therefore, proper growth and development is not achieved by the child. By observing this, the Vāgbhaṭa has mentioned that in these children attainment of youth is doubtful.

Features of unconscious (asphyxiated) baby

(As mentioned by Vāgbhaṭa (A.S.U. 1/3)

* Deep unconsciousness

** No cry (even after deep stimulation)

*** Decreased or unstable dhātus

**** Hypersensitivity of pain stimuli

***** Dieing like appearance.

Methods of resuscitation, mentioned for normal as well as asphyxiated newborn, by Caraka and Suśruta are their original contributions, however, Suśruta has made slight change in sequence of various steps of resuscitation. Other Āyurvedic texts have followed Caraka. Vedic literature has not given specific description regarding the management (resuscitation) of newborn. It looks very surprising that various steps of resuscitation mentioned by ancient scholars, thousands year before; are practised even today by modern pediatricians with slight modifications.

During the process of resuscitation, production of sound by two stones may stimulate the newborn through auditary stimulation, while sprinkling of hot/cold water may produce sensory stimulation. The reflexes of these stimulations may ultimately stimulate the cardio-respiratory functions. Lipton et al. (1966) have established the fact that the neonate can discriminate sound on the basis of frequency, intensity and stimulus dimensionality. A low frequency stimulus tends to have a soothing effect on the neonate, whereas a high frequency stimulus causes an immediate arousal. As the sound is localised, cardiac rate first increases and may be accompanied by a mild startle.

Features of an unconscious (asphyxiated) newborn baby, as mentioned by Vāgbhaṭa have quite resemblance with APGAR Scoring used now-a-days for assessing the status of asphyxiated baby. By observing the features, described by Vāgbhaṭa, one can assess the condition and outcome of newborn (asphyxiated). Actually the features mentioned by Vāgbhaṭa, are different stages of hypoxia, and its specific explanation may be given very well. Deep unconsciousness, absence of cry and dieing like appearance are the features of severe asphyxia. Severely asphyxiated newborn is either deeply stuporous or in coma. He has marked hypotonia or flaccidity and exhibits little spontaneous limb movement. Infant does not cry on painful stimulation.

Descreased or unstable dhātus can be referred for poor oxygenation of blood and/or poor cardiac output, due to cardio-respiratory failure in asphyxiated newborn.

Hypersensitivity of pain stimuli is a feature of moderate hypoxia. This stage have definite signs including irritability, vomiting, increased muscle tone and a high-pitched poorly sustained cry.

According to Vāgbhaṭa the above features may also manifest in hyperpyrexia. In newborn, common cause of hyperpyrexia is septicemia, which may present various features including above signs.

(c) *Cutting and care of umbilical cord*

During intra-uterine life, baby receives its nutrition from mother through umbilical cord. After birth, placenta is separated from mother, therefore cutting of umbilical cord becomes necessary, just after delivery. Improper cutting of cord may cause various complications.

Most of the Āyurvedic texts have given appropriate description of cutting and care of umbilical cord. Caraka opines that after measuring the cord 8 angulas (app. 4") from the umbilicus, it is hold with two fingers and to be cut with the ardha-dhārāśastra (knife). This instrument should be made of gold, silver, iron or of any other metal. The cut end of the cord should be tied properly with thread and hanged loosely with the neck.[23] However, Suśruta is of opinion that umbilical cord at first should be tied at the 8 angulas distance and then it should be cut and tied in the neck of the baby.[24] Ḍalhaṇa, while commenting, has explained that hanging of umbilical cord in the neck will prevent the oozing of blood from it. The cord should be irrigated properly with Kuṣṭha Taila.[25]

Other authors of Āyurvedic texts[26] and Ugrādityācārya, the author of a Jain book Kalyāṇa Kāraka,[27] have followed the views of Caraka and Suśruta. However, Vāgbhaṭa has advised that umbilical cord should be cut only four angulas distal to umbilicus.

The length of umbilical cord, as described by Caraka and Suśruta seems to be much long, because it may cause inconvenience to the baby, however, the length described by Vāgbhaṭa (4 angulas) appears to be appropriate.

Suśruta, at one place, is quite right that cord should be cut only after tieing, while Caraka and others have advised first to cut then to tie. This practice may cause much bleeding from the cord. Tieing of umbilical cord in the neck of baby may be good for certain reasons—protection from injury, decreasing the chances of leaking of blood due to anti-gravity position, and reducing the chances of contamination from urine and stool.

2. General Care of Infant

General nursing care of newborn includes bath, feeding (nutrition and fluid intake), clothings, maintenance of body temperature and protection from infections.

(a) *Bath*

Suśruta opines that after delivery the baby should be massaged with Balā-taila. Bath should be given, keeping in view the kāla (period), vitiation or influence of doṣas and bala (strength) of the child. Bath should be given with luke-warm decoction of Kṣīrī-vṛkṣa (latex yielding plants) or luke-warm sarvagandhodaka or with luke-warm water treated with heated gold or silver rod or with luke-warm decoction of leaves of Kapittha.[28]

Ḍalhaṇa has mentioned specific conditions for the use of different types of water (medicated), which are as follows:[29]

	Type of water	*Condition*
1.	Decoction of kṣīrī-vṛkṣa	Dominance of pitta
2.	Sarvagandhodaka	Dominance of vāta
3.	Hot water prepared by immersing heated gold or silver rod	Less strength of baby
4.	Decoction of kapittha leaves	Less strength of baby

Vāgbhaṭa[30] and compiler of Yogaratna Samuccaya[31] have followed Suśruta, however, Bhoja (Rāj Martaṇḍa)[32] have mentioned a different procedure of bath. Before bath decoction of leaves of Saptcchada (Satwan), Arka and roots of Naktamāla, Karañja mixed with cow's urine, should be anointed on whole body then the bath should be given, with water prepared with Netrabālā and Muṇḍī.

(b) *Feeding for first 4 days*

Newborn, after birth, is totally dependent on oral feeding. Although mother milk is best for babies but during first few days (1-4 days), most of mothers do not have sufficient secretion of milk. Ancient scholars were very much aware of this fact, that is why they have specifically prescribed feeding schedule of neonate from 1st to 4th day after birth.

Caraka is of the opinion that on 1st day of birth, baby should be offered honey and ghṛta as first feed and from next feed, right breast should be offered for sucking.[33] Suśruta[34] and Vāgbhaṭa[35] have given different feeding schedule. On first day honey and ghṛta mixed with Anantā in baby's palmful quantity, consecrated with mantras should be given to newborn, thrice a day. On second and third day, ghṛta medicated with Laxmaṇā is to be given. On 4th day madhu (honey) and ghṛta should be offered two times in the day (morning and noon) and from evening onward breast feeding should be started.

Buddhist literature has prescribed butter as first feed after giving first bath to newborn.[36] In 'Mūla Sārvastivāda,' in reference to the birth of Jīvaka, there is description to offer honey and ghṛta.[37]

Table-1: Feeding schedule for neonate from first to fourth day after birth

Day	*C.S.*	*S.S.*	*A.S.*	*A.H.*	*Buddhist Litt.* *Divyā.*	*Mūla.*
Ist day	Madhu + Ghṛta + Breast milk	Madhu + Ghṛta + Anantā	Madhu + Ghṛta + Anantā	Madhu + Ghṛta + Anantā	Butter	Madhu & Ghṛta
2nd day	Breast milk	Madhu + Ghṛta + Laxmaṇā	Madhu + Ghṛta + Laxmaṇā	madhu + Ghṛta + Laxmaṇā	-	-
3rd day	-do-	-do-	-do-	-do-	-do-	-do-
4th day upto noon	-do-	-do-	-do-	Butter	-	-
evening	-do-	Breast milk	Breast milk	Breast milk		

The opinion of Caraka to provide breast milk on 1st day, seems to be appropriate that most of the mothers can provide breast feed to their babies. But on the other hand Suśruta is also right on his views because practically there may be delay in milk secretion, especially in primiparous mothers and it may take about 2-3 days to set proper milk secretion. Therefore, an alternative feeding schedule must be prescribed, which the Suśruta and followers have mentioned. But it look very surprising that ancient scholars except Caraka, have not considered the importance of fluid requirement of the newborn in first 3 days while it is very important at this stage, however, it is possible that unwritten instructions to give water as per requirement might be provided.

(c) *Cloths and bed*

Caraka has described various qualities of bed and cloths. Suśruta has advised that the baby should be wrapped with soft cloths.[38] Baby bed should also have soft cloths. According to Vāgbhaṭa, the baby should be made to sleep on a cushion made of soft cloths, keeping the head on east side.[39] Buddhist literature advises to use white cloths.[40]

(d) *Protective measures (Rakṣā karma)*

The following measures were advocated by various ancient scholars, to protect the newborn from influence of various evil powers (infections).

Measures advised by Caraka[41]

1. The twigs of Ādanī, Khadira, Karkandhu, Pīlu and Parūṣaka should be hanged and Sarṣapa, Atasī, Taṇḍula and Kaṇakaṇīka should be strewn around and inside of Sūtikāgāra (maternity room).
2. Taṇḍula bali oblation should be performed in morning and evening for ten days.
3. A wooden pestle (mūsala) should be placed over door-sill in oblique position.
4. Various rakṣoghna (bacteriostatic/bacteriocidal) drugs like Vacā, Kuṣṭha, Kṣaumaka, Hingu, Sarṣapa, Atasī, Laśuna, Kaṇakaṇīyaka and Guggulu, etc. are kept in a packet and hanged in the upper portion of door-frame.

Small packets containing these above drugs should also be tied in the neck of the puerperal woman and newborn, over cooking pot, pots filled with water, bed and on both the pannets of door.

5. Inside the Sūtikāgāra, fire should be lit daily with the woods of Kaṇakakaṇṭaka or Tinduka.

6. The attendents present in Sūtikāgāra should remain awaken for 10 or 12 days to take special care of the mother and newborn.

7. Śānti-homa should be performed daily in morning and evening, by the Brāhmaṇas, possessing knowledge of Atharva Veda.

Measures advised by Suśruta:[42]

1. Baby should be fanned with twigs of Pīlu, Badrī, Nimba and Parūṣaka.

2. Tampoon soaked in oil should be applied over head.

3. Fumigation with rakṣoghna drugs (Vacā, etc.) should be done and small packets made of these drugs should be tied in arms, legs, head and neck of the newborn.

4. Tila, Atasī, Sarṣapa and Kaṇā should be scattered all around.

5. Measures prescribed for wounded person, in other chapter of the book, may be taken into consideration for use, if necessary.

Measures advised by Vāgbhaṭa:[43]

1. The fanning by the twigs of various drugs like Ādārī, Vidārī, Badarī, Khadir, Nimba, Pīlu and Parūṣaka should be done on baby. These drugs should be also scattered all around Sūtikāgāra. Other drugs like Sarṣapa, Atasī and Kaṇakaṇika, etc. should be scattered outside as well as inside of the house.

2. Dhūpan should be done by Guggulu, Aguru, Sarjarasa and Gaura Sarṣapa.

3. Śānti karma should be done for 10 days. For this purpose recitation of Māyurī, Mahāmāyūrī, Āryā, Ratnaketu, Dhāriṇī, should be done twice a day.
4. Small packets, containing Hingu, Vacā and Turūṣaka should be tied in the head and neck of the child.

Bhūrja-patra having inscription of hymn like Parṇasabarī, Āryā, Aprājitā written with gorocana, should be tied in the head and neck of the child.

Other texts including Caraka have given few other measures to protect the child, but these are seems to be of use for later period of childhood, therefore, described in other chapter (General Care of Children).

Care of Child on Saṣṭhī Rātri (Sixth Night of Birth)

Literature of 5-6 century A.D. have description about the special care of child on the 6th night of his birth.

Vāgbhaṭa has advised that on 6th night of birth of the child, all the family members and friends remain awaken and rakṣā-karma should be performed by offering sacrifices.[44]

Bāṇa Bhatta, writer of Kādambarī, has mentioned about the birth of Candrapīḍa and the description of care of baby on sixth night.[45]

Most of the drugs prescribed for the protection purpose have anti-septic properties. It is very interesting to note that ancient scholars have observed very closely about the most crucial period of infancy and marked it upto six days. Care of 6th night indicate that from birth to 6th days period, babies are most susceptible to various infections (tetanus neonatorum etc.) and other complications. After one week, the incidence of infections and complications reduce, therefore, the chance of survival increase. Provision of putting pot filled with water may probably solve the purpose to maintain humidity in Kumārāgāra (Nursery).

REFERENCES

1. C.S.Śā. 4.25; S.S.Śā. 3.16; A.S.Śā. 2.30; A.H.Śā. 1.66; K.S.Śā. 4.1
2. A.V.I. 11.1
3. A.V.I. 11.2
4. A.V.I. 11.3
5. A.V.I. 11.4
6. A.V.I. 11.5
7. A.V.I. 11.6
8. A.V.I. 11.7
9. A.V.VI. 110.2-3
10. Divyā. 18. page 146
11. C.S.Śā.8. 42-46
12. S.S.Śā. 10.11,12
13. A.S.Śā. 3.37; A.S.U. 1.2, 3, 5-10
14. A.H.U. 1.1, 2, 5-11
15. K.K. 18.29
16. C.D. 64.3
17. Y.R.S. 22.321
18. C.D. 64.3
19. Mārkaṇḍeya Pu. 11.18
20. C.S.Śā. 8.42
21. A.S.U. 1,3,4
22. A.S.U. 1.4; A.H.U. 1.3,4
23. C.S.Śā. 8.44
24. S.S.Śā. 10.11
25. S.S.Śā. 10.11 Ḍalhaṇa Comm.
26. A.S.U. 1.5; A.H.U. 1.5,6; Y.R.S. 22.322, 323(1)
27. K.K. 18.29
28. S.S.Śā. 10.12
29. S.S.Śā. 10.12 Ḍalhaṇa Comm.

30. A.S.U. 1.6; A.H.U. 1.6, 7
31. Y.R.S. 22.323(2), 324, 325
32. R.M. Bāl. 14
33. C.S.Śā. 8.46
34. S.S.Śā. 10.14
35. A.S.U. 1.12, 13; A.H.U. 1.12-14
36. Divyā. 35. page 427
37. Mūla Sarvā. 1, 2. page 183
38. S.S.Śā. 10.20
39. A.S.U. 1.14,15
40. Divyā. 35. page 427
41. C.S.Śā. 8.47
42. S.S.Śā. 10.20
43. A.S.U. 1.16-19
44. A.S.U.1.26; A.H.U. 1.21
45. Kādambarī (Pūrva) page 229.

2

Infant Feeding

Food is one of the basic needs of human life. The nutritional problems of childhood differ from those of adults. All nutrients must provide not only energy and replacement of tissue, but also for growth involving an increase in size of all tissues in the body. Growth has its highest rate of increase in infancy. Thus nutritional problems are most liable to occur during this period. Therefore, it is very essential to take proper care of child for nutrition.

Keeping in view, the above facts, ancient literature of Āyurveda have classified the childhood period on the basis of their food requirement, i.e., Kṣīrapa (milk is main diet) upto one year; Kṣīrānnāda (milk and cereals both) from 1-2 years; and Annāda[1] (cereals as main diet) two years onwards. This indicate that ancient scholars were very much aware of feeding of children, especially for infants. Initially milk is only main feed, therefore, much stress has been put forth for describing various aspects of milk.

Milk

Milk is the main and primary diet of children. Breast feeding was considered very excellent food for infants, even in Vedic period. Ṛg Veda has advocated breast feeding after birth with recitation of mantras. Skanda, mentioned in dharma granthas became popular as 'Kārtikeya,' only because of being breast fed by six 'Kṛttikās.'[2] This reference reflects the importance of breast milk.

Caraka considered milk a wholesome diet, as it provides full nutrition, increases strength and keeps one healthy.[3] Suśruta has elaborated the views of Caraka and said that milk is very first and natural diet of all the animals including human beings. In general state of body, milk provides strength, it is aphrodisiac and also increases immunity, while in diseased state it is congenial and also helpful in keeping doṣas in balanced state.[4] Kaśyapa has expressed similar view like Caraka and Suśruta.[5] Hārīta has explained role of milk in keeping a person free from various ailments and mentioned that milk purifies sṛotasas, keeps doṣas in balanced state and increases appetite and improves digestion.[6]

Breast Milk

Breast milk is best food for infants. Caraka opines that it provides vitality and is anabolic (Bramhaṇa) wholesome (Sātmya) and unctuous (Snigdha). It is also useful as a nasal drops in Rakta Pitta and for eye diseases, as instillation.[7] Along with various physiological properties, Suśruta[8] has mentioned physical properties of breast milk. Breast milk is sweet but Kaṣāya (astringent) in anurasa (secondary taste), cold in nature, vivifying, laghu (light) and appetiser. He further gives instruction that breast milk should never be heated. Vāgbhaṭa and other scholars opine that child grow properly on breast feeding.[9] Hārīta has mentioned the properties of breast milk similar to Caraka,[10] however, he has given very interesting description that the properties of breast milk may change according to complexion of woman (mother).[11]

1. Milk of black complexioned mother — nutritious and pacifies vāta.

2. White complexioned mother — increases kapha.
3. Yellowish complexioned mother — pacifies pitta.

Milk of blackish and yellowish complexioned mother have been considered better.

Concepts of ancient scholars are very well supported by modern medical science, however, modern science has given various advantages of breast milk, while ancients have concentrated mainly on the maintenance of body and prevention of various ailments. It means that they were very well aware of nutritive and immunological values of breast milk.

Human milk is the most appropriate of all available other milks for infants. Breast milk is always readily available at the proper temperature and no time is required for preparation. The milk is fresh and free from contamination, so chances of gastrointestinal disturbances are negligible. Human milk also contains bacterial and viral antibodies, including relatively high concentrations of secretory Ig A antibodies.

Formation and Secretion of Milk

In sequence of description of formation of dhātus, Caraka has mentioned that milk is produced from rasa dhātu.[12] However, Suśruta has clarified the process of milk formation and mentioned that food after proper digestion and assimilation changes in the form of rasa dhātu and purest form of it converts into milk, after reaching in breasts. For easy understanding the process of lactation, Suśruta has given example of Śukra. In normal state of body, as Śukra remain pervaded in whole of the body but remembrance, touching of her body parts or intercourse, it collects in Śukrāśaya and ejaculate from penis. In the same way, like Śukra, milk also secretes with the stimulation of mother due to following factors:[13]

1. By touching of her body by the child.
2. Looking the child.
3. Remembrance of the child.
4. Keeping child in her lap.
5. Touching of her breast by the child.

The chief factor, among the above, is affection of mother to her child.[14]

After 3-4 days of birth, dhamanīs (milk carrying channels) of the woman open and secretion of milk starts.

Concepts of Suśruta regarding lactation process is very much scientific. In fact affection of mother to the child is an important factor, responsible for production and ejection of breast milk. Secretion of milk depends on various reflexes, described in modern texts.

Kaśyapa has also considered that milk is a by-product of rasa dhātu. During pregnancy, the rasa dhātu performs three functions:[15]

1. Nutrition of woman herself
2. Nutrition of fetus, and
3. Formation of milk.

However, Kaśyapa has also considered that rakta-dhātu play a role in formation of milk.[16(a)] Describing process for formation of milk, Kaśyapa has given the example of cow as follow:[16(b)]

In ancient time, by churning of ocean, nectar appeared as a essence of all Auṣadhis, Milk is also formed in the same way after reaching of āhāra in the abdomen of cows.

Vāgbhaṭa and Ācārya Mādhava are of the same opinion like Suśruta:[17]

Hārīta Saṃhitā has raised two queries:[18]

1. How the colour of milk become white, while the colour of blood is red?

2. Why there is no milk formation in virgins and infertile women?

While answering the first question Ātreya has explained that initially milk remain concentrated and red but after maturation by pitta, its colour become white. Thus ultimately, the colour of milk is white.

The main cause due to which milk formation does not occur, is related with the nāḍi, responsible for formation of milk. Due to deficiency of proper dhātu (hormones) in virgins, nāḍis responsible for milk formation are not properly developed. While in case of infertile women the milk producing nāḍis, remain blocked by Vāyu, causing failure in milk formation but formation of ārtava occur in large amount.

In woman, the child delivers with force. By this force srotasas open up and lactation starts. Milk of a newly parous woman is Kaphaja, so it is more thick (concentrated). Probably due to this reason the writer has contraindicated the use of this milk.[19]

Kālidāsa, in the text Kumāra Sambhavam has also considered the psychological factor, responsible for lactation.[20]

Though apparently it looks that there is difference of opinion regarding formation of stanya (breast milk), because it is described to be formed from rasa and rakta. Prof. Tewari in her book (Āyurvedīya Prasūti Tantra) has clarified it very well and explained very scientifically that during pregnancy new lactic glands and lactiferous tubules are formed, existing grow and develop. For growth and development, during pregnancy period the rakta (blood) is essential, first milk secretion or colostrum is also formed during pregnancy from rakta. After delivery there is no further growth of lactic glands, but their function, i.e., formation of milk is increased, which is accomplished by rasa.

Properties and Examination of Pure Milk

The child should always be provided only pure (normal) breast milk, because vitiated (abnormal) milk can produce various disorders in the child. Caraka has described properties and examinations of pure (normal) milk, according to its physical properties. The normal milk must be of natural colour, smell, taste and touch, and should be mixed completely in water. Normal (pure) milk provides health and strength.[21] However, Caraka has not mentioned the natural colour of milk. But Suśruta opines that pure milk must be Pāṇḍura (yellowish white) in colour and madhura (sweet) in taste.[22]

Following test should be done to detect the purity of milk:

Milk on pouring in a vessel, containing water, should possess following findings:[23]

1. Dissolves very well in water.
2. No appearance of foam.
3. No fibrous appearance.
4. Neither it flows nor it settles down.

Contrary to Caraka and Suśruta, Kaśyapa has decided purity of milk according to its effects on body. Normal milk should possess following properties:[24]

1. Natural and pure milk is cold, clear, thin and resemble with the colour of Konch shell (Śankhāvabhāsa).
2. It provides strength to the child and his growth is proper.
3. It produces no harm to the child and even to the mother.

Most of the treatises of later period have mentioned the water taste of milk for observing its purity and all are of one opinion regarding the following facts:[25]

1. Pure milk on pouring in water, mixes very well in it.
2. Child develops and grows satisfactorily without having any complication.

Dhātrī (Wet-Nurse)

Mother milk has been considered very useful and nutritious to the child right from ancient period. However, if due to any circumstances, mother milk is not available, a woman was arranged to feed her breast to the child. These women were named 'dhātrī.' Ancient literature has sufficient references of dhātrī.

According to Caraka[26] a dhātrī should be considered fit for breast feeding, only when she have following qualities:

1. She should be of similar caste to that of chilid.
2. She should be young, reliable and disease free (healthy).
3. Her body parts should be in proper form. She should be free from bad habits, should not be ugly and badly dressed.
4. Dhātrī and child should be of similar place.
5. She should be born in a reputed family. Neither she nor her work should be of low mentality.
6. She should have affection for the child and her own children must be alive. Mentally she should be healthy.
7. She should be able to produce sufficient quantity of milk.
8. She should not sleep too much and should be very alert in the service of child.
9. She should follow the rules of religion and should also take care of hygiene.
10. Her breast should be healthy having secretion of good quality of milk.

Breast having following qualities are considered good:

Breast should not be too high, too long, too thin and much longer. The shape of the nipples should be proper, so that the child can suck properly.

Suśruta,[27] while describing the qualities of good dhātrī, has described almost similar properties like Caraka and has stressed on two factors—i.e., complexion of dhātrī and qualities of breasts. He considers that a dhātrī having dark complexion (śyāma) is good. Any defect in the breast may produce various abnormalities in the child. If a dhātrī having too high breasts, the child become with big protending teeth (Karālamukha), on sucking such breasts. Large breasts may cover the mouth and nostrils of child and ultimately death may occur.

Modern views have very well clarified this concept of Suśruta. Elizabet Helsing (1984) writes that an infant may seem to gag and choke, if the nipple is long that it goes past the hard palate and touches the soft palate. It may react by fighting, when put to the breast, it turns its head, cries and moves its arms and legs. This can easily be corrected by holding the infant little away from the breast.

Suśruta has advocated that dhātrī, once appointed should not be changed too frequently, because by doing so, the child receives the milk of different qualities. This practice is not congenial for child and he may suffer from various disorders, therefore, it is advisable to appoint only one dhātrī for nursing the child.[28] Suśruta further mentions that there are certain conditions in which dhātrī should not offer her breasts to the child. Such conditions are—hunger, sadness, anger, with vitiated dhātus, pregnancy, following various diet (āhāras) and mode of life (vihāras) which are antagonistic in action. If dhātrī has received any medicine then breast feeding should also be avoided until the effect of medicine has passed off.[29]

In Kaśyapa Saṃhitā, there is description of dhātrī milk. Methods for increasing the quantity and purification of milk are described in this chapter. This Chapter is interrupted in the beginning, therefore, it is possible that missing part may contain the description of dhātrī.

Kaśyapa has praised dhātrī—'Dhātrī due to her affection with child ruins her body. She bears many griefs, hope, affection, mercy, etc. for care of her child and feels proud.'[30]

Vāgbhaṭa has also mentioned various qualities of dhātrī and also advised to discard the dhātrī having Aṣṭa-doṣas of body like—too short, too tall, too dark, too fair (complexion), too hairy, without hairs, too obese or too thin (weak). Her nipples should not be too much directed towards downward or upward and should not be of very small or large size.[31] Description of defects of breasts is similar like Suśruta, however, Vāgbhaṭa has restricted the use of milk of pregnant dhātrī. The child may suffer from Pārigarbhika disease on consuming such type of milk.[32]

In Aṣṭānga Hṛdaya, Vāgbhaṭa has advised to appoint two dhātrīs, in non-availability of mother milk.[33]

The word 'Dhātī' is found in Pali language.[34] It's duty is said to take care of child and feed in absence of mother milk. In Buddhist period, there was provision of appointing four types of dhātrīs.[35]

1. Dhātrī for breast feeding (Khīram pāyenti)
2. Dhātrī for giving bath (Nhāpeti)
3. Dhātrī for general nursing care (Dhārenti)
4. Dhātrī for holding baby in her lap (Ankena Pariharandi)

In Mūgapakkha Jātaka (No. 538),[36] qualities of good dhātrī are described. In the story, it has been mentioned that the king of Varanasi has appointed 500 dhātrīs for care of his son. In the same story defects of dhātrī and its effect on the child are mentioned.

	Defects of dhātrī	*Effect on child*
1.	Too long	neck become much longer
2.	Too short	drooped shoulder
3.	Too thin	pain in thighs
4.	Too healthy (fatty)	bow-legged

Jain literature has mentioned about five types of dhātrī, for nursing of child.[37] These are—Kṣīra dhātrī, Majjana dhātrī, Maṇḍana dhātrī, Kṛīḍana dhātrī and Anka dhātrī.

1. Kṣīra dhātrī—Colour of Kṣīra dhātrī should be similar to that of child. In general, dhātrī of dark complexion (śyāmā) has been considered good, while milk of dhātrī having black complexion has not been considered good. The breast milk of the dhātrī, having whitish complexion has been considered of less strength.
2. Majjana dhātrī—The work of this dhātrī is to keep the child clean.
3. Maṇḍana dhātrī—The duty of maṇḍana dhātrī is to dress the child.
4. Kṛīḍana dhātrī—She plays with child. Her voice and personality affect the child. Kṛīdana dhātrī having harmonious voice has been considered good. The duty of this dhātrī is also to care the child from Pūtanā.
5. Anka dhātrī—Any defect of anka dhātrī may affect the child. The child may be of deformed foot if she is fatty; feels uncomfortable if she is lean and thin and may develop shy behaviour if dhātrī is of rough hands.

In ancient India, tradition of appointing dhātrī in non-availability of mother milk, is inimitable. Such great importance of it was not given in any other part of the world, except in Egypt, where the use of a wet-nurse (dhātrī) for infant feeding began first in the Ptolemaic period (4th century B.C.), through Greek influence.

Most of the description of dhātrī is available in Āyurvedic text, Buddhist and Jain literature. Most of the scholars, have considered that any dhātrī should have following qualities:

1. Physical—good health, young/middle age, capable of producing sufficient quantity of milk, having breast of proper shape and size.
2. Mental—affection with child.
3. Habit—alert, free from bad habits.
4. Social—belongs to reputed family.

Suśruta has praised dhātrī of dark complexion (śyāmā). Jain literature has also considered that dhātrī of dark complexion is good, while milk of such (dark complexion) dhatrī has not been considered good. Its proper explanation appears to be very difficult.

Appointment of more than one dhātrī was prevalent probably in royal families, however, concept of dhātrī, in ancient period, indicate the awareness of infant feeding, especially of breast feeding.

Method of Breast Feeding

Ṛg Veda advocated to offer breast milk after birth, with recitation of mantras.[38] Caraka has advised that before performing Jātakarma, the child should be offered madhu and ghṛta and then with the same process, right breast should be offered first, with recitation of mantras.[39] But before offering breast, dhātrī should take bath properly, anoint herself with Candana and wear white garments, she should tie all or available drugs out of—Aindrī, Brāhmī, Śatvīryā, Sahasravīryā, Amoghā, Avyathā, Śivā, Ariṣṭā, Vātyapuṣpī and Viṣvaksena kāṇṭā. Dhātrī should sit facing towards east and then offer her right breast first.[40]

Suśruta has given similar method of breast feeding with some differences and opines that feeding should be started from auspicious day time. Before offering first feed, the child should be given bath and new garments to wear. The dhātrī should sit facing towards east and hold the child in her lap, keeping his face to the north side, then breast feeding should be offered with enchanting of mantras.[41]

In his description Suśruta has mentioned a special point which must be kept always in mind of dhātrī. While offering breast feed, dhātrī should discard some amount of milk from her breasts, before giving to the child. If this fact is over ruled then the child may suffer from Kāsa, Śvāsa, Vaman, etc. due to blockade of sṛotasas of breast.[42]

Vāgbhaṭa has also advised similar method of breast feeding like Suśruta and mentioned that at the time of breast feeding dhātrī should be cheerful and should tie various drugs like Aindrī, Dūrvā, etc. Prajāsthāpanī drugs. Vāgbhaṭa has given different explanation for discarding some milk before breast feeding and opines that due to fullness of breasts, milk suddenly come out of the breast and produces complications.[43] Modern scientists also have similar explanation. Elisabet Helsing (1984) mentions that when a mother has too much milk ejection reflex, the milk fills the infants mouth too quickly and chokes it. To avoid the situation, mother should express some milk before the infant feed. One thing is also very interesting to note that most of the ancient scholars have advocated that breast feeding should be offered in sitting position. This position of mother and child will help to remove swallowed air, thus preventing regurgitation of milk.

Milk, Prescribed in Non-Availability of Breast Milk

It is well accepted fact that breast milk is congenial to children, but if, due to circumstances breast milk is not available then one should prescribe the milk to the child which is similar to that of breast milk. Most of the ancient scholars are of opinion that milk of cow and goat has very much resemblance with breast milk, both in composition and properties.

Vāgbhaṭa, in the text Aṣṭānga Hṛdaya, has also advocated the milk of goat or cow in non-availability of breast milk, but it should be given after treating with drugs of Laghu Pañcamūla or only by Śālaparṇī and Pṛśnaparṇī.[44]

Āyurvedic texts have given description of 8 types of milk. These are—milk of women, cow's milk, goat's milk, buffalo's milk, ass's milk or horse's milk, sheep's milk, camel's milk and elephant's milk. Out of these only goat's and cow's milk have been prescribed in non-availability of breast milk[45] as these have similar properties with mother milk, therefore, references of cow's and goat's milk are recapitulated here.

Cow's Milk: Caraka has considered that after breast milk, cow's milk is better. It possess following properties—Svādu (tasty), śīta (vīrya), mṛdu (soft), snigdha (unctuous), bahala (thick), ślakṣṇa (soft), picchila (slimy), guru (heavy), manḍa and prasanna (clear).[46]

These above said properties of cow's milk have resemblance with oja (vital power). Therefore, use of cow's milk will certainly increase the oja. Due to this fact cow's milk has been considered superior to all other food articles and have Jīvanīya property. Suśruta has also considered it abhiṣyandī, snigdha, guru, rasāyana, raktapitta nāśaka, śītala, madhura (in pāka), increases longevity and cures the disorders of vāta and pitta.

Kaśyapa has described the properties of cow's milk in a different way. According to him properties of cow's milk depend upon the articles, which she (cow) consumes, because, milk is ultimately formed from the diet. Cow usually consume the diet which is madhura and lavaṇa in nature, therefore, milk produced by them is also madhura.[47] Madhura rasa is considered to have vṛṃhaṇa and rasāyana effects.

Vāgbhaṭa is of similar opinion and considered that cow's milk is jīvanīya, rasāyana, medhā vardhaka (helpful in restoring intelligence) and bala vardhaka (increases strength). Therapeutically it is also useful in convalescence, giddiness, respiratory disorders, excessive thirst, hunger, chronic fever, dysurea and haemorrhagic disorders.[48]

Hārīta has given very interesting description of properties of cow's milk. According to him properties of milk changes according to the colour of cow and considered that fresh (dhāroṣṇa) milk is better.[49]

According to modern knowledge the composition of breast milk varies during each feed, in the course of the day, in the course of lactation, between different women and even in the same woman between the two breasts and in different pregnancies.

Breast and cow's milk have a similar energy content but cow's milk contains three times the amount of protein and much less lactose and fat than breast milk. The protein in cow's milk is mainly casein, whereas in breast milk a greater proportion is lactalbumin and whey protein. The electrolytes, sodium, potassium, calcium and chloride all occur in cow's milk in about 3 to 4 times the concentration in breast milk and the mean phosphorous content is 6 times as much. In order to reduce the amount of protein and electrolytes, cow's milk is usually diluted before being fed to babies and sugar added to return the energy value to about 700 K Cal/L.

Lavin et al. (1950) found no difference in serum protein in full term or pre-term infants but weight gain of pre-term infants on breast milk was lower than on cow's milk and they suggested that this might be due to high protein contents of cow's milk.

Cow's milk should be offered to the child, after proper boiling it, because bovine tuberculosis may affect the child, if taken without boiling.

Goat's Milk: Caraka opines that goat's milk is astringent and sweet (in rasa), cold (in vīrya) and light. It solidifies stool. It also cures haemorrhagic disorders, diarrhoea, tuberculosis, cough and fever.[50] Suśruta has considered that it has similar properties to cow's milk. It is easily digestable and congenial in various disorders. Goat has comparatively smaller body, eats leaves of plants which are bitter, drink little amount of water and usually wander, thus their milk is congenial in all type of disorders.[51]

Kaśyapa has mentioned properties of goat's milk in the similar way, which have been described by previous scholars like Caraka and Suśruta. However, he has the concept that goat's milk is more concentrated because it is secreted in less quantity and is Vṛṃhaṇa (due to concentration).[52]

Vāgbhaṭa has followed Suśruta while Hārīta to the all previous scholars.[53]

Although goat's milk is similar in composition to cow's milk. However, it contains less sodium, more potassium and chloride, and more of the essential linoleic and arachidonic acids. It's fat may be more digestable and it's curd tension is lower than that found in cow's milk. It is low in vitamin D, iron and folic acid. Infants fed exclusively on goat's milk are prone to megaloblastic anemia due to folate deficiency. The goat is especially susceptible to brucellosis, therefore, milk should be boiled before use.

Since time immemorial till today, there is no basic change in concept of feeding and nutrition of the newborn and infant. Mother milk is superior to all other food articles. In certain circumstances mother milk may be replaced or supplemented by cow's milk. This is fact that there is no other best alternative to it. Methods described in ancient time are still highly useful and acceptable to all.

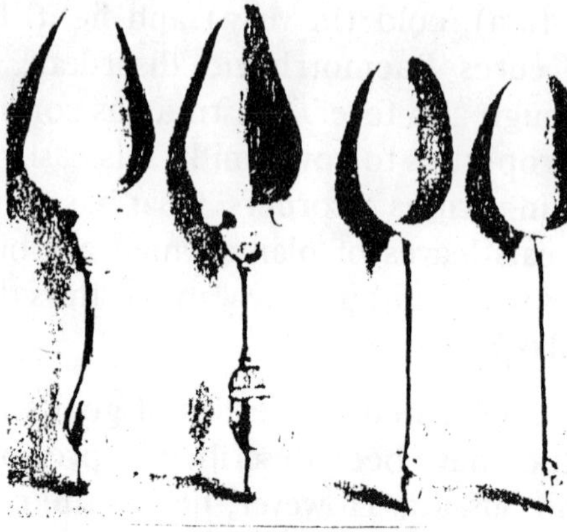

Plate 1—Iron Spoons Used for Feeding (1st Century AD)

Weaning (Introduction of Cereals)

In fact, breast feeding is a good diet for children, however, with increasing the age, nutritional requirements also increases and only milk cannot fulfil the requirement. Therefore, it becomes essential to introduce other food articles to them. References from ancient literature indicate that ancient scholars were aware of this fact.

Caraka has not given any specific description of weaning. Suśruta and Vāgbhaṭa have advised that weaning should be started from 6th month of age while Kaśyapa has advised that at the age of 6th month, the child should be offered fruit juice and semi-solid food from the age of 10th month.[54]

Food articles used for weaning: In ancient period, following food articles or recipes, were used for weaning purpose:

1. In Pāraskara Gṛhya Sūtra,[55] a simple principle has been followed that food of all kinds and of different sort of flavours should be mixed together and given to the child.

Most of the Gṛhya Sūtras[56] have advocated the use of flesh of various birds and other food articles for weaning. Weaning foods have it's effect on the child.

	Food articles	*Effect on child*
(i)	Flesh of bird Bhārdvāja	Fluency of speech
(ii)	Flesh of bird Kapiñjala and ghṛta	Proper nourishment
(iii)	Flesh of bird Kṛkasa or rice mixed with honey	Long life
(iv)	Flesh of bird Ati	Holy lustere
(v)	Rice mixed with ghṛta	Brilliance
(vi)	Curd and rice	Strong senses.

2. Suśruta has advised that the food (cereals) used for weaning must be easy to digest (laghu).[57]
3. Flesh of birds like Lāvaka, Kapiñjala, Tittara, Carṇāyudha (cock) are advised by Kaśyapa, for weaning.[58]
4. Vāgbhaṭa mentioned the description of modaka made of Priyāla, Madhuyaṣṭī, Madhu, Lājā and Sugar-candy should be given to children.

Description of one another modaka (sweet-balls) is also mentioned which are made of unripened fruits of Bilva, Elā, Sugar and Lājā (parched paddy).[59] These stimulates appetite and provides nutrition.

Vāgbhaṭa has advised a method by which a mother can divert the attention of child from breast feeding so that the child may take other food articles, which are provided to him. For this purpose, mother should show less affection with the child, make her breast hideous by applying leethsome anointment and making artificial wound by applying Alaktaka. By seeing such type of breast, child will refuse to suck. The quantity of food article should be increased and milk should be decreased gradually.[60]

Various lehas mentioned by Kaśyapa,[61] may also be introduced to children as weaning because these are indicated in the conditions in which mother have not adequate secretion of breast milk or she is unfit for providing her breasts due to her illness or vitiation of milk. These lehas are also described for increasing medhā (intellect) and providing immunity to the children, therefore, are discussed in detail in other chapter 'General Care of Children.'

Causes of Inadequate Milk Secretion (Stanya-Nāśa)

The child grows properly, if his mother/dhātrī provides him breast milk in sufficient quantity. But due to certain conditions, secretion of milk becomes less, and ultimately, the child may suffer from various nutritional disorders.

Caraka has not mentioned any specific cause, responsible for cessation of milk secretion, however, while describing the drugs for increasing milk secretion, he has restricted the consumption of Sīdhu (a type of wine). It means that use of Sīdhu may reduce the milk secretion.[62]

Suśruta has stressed mainly on psychological factors, responsible for cessation of milk secretion and mentioned that if dhātri is angry, grieved and has less affection with the child; will reduce her milk secretion.[63]

Kaśyapa opines that cessation of milk secretion may be due to nature (Svabhāva). Some other factors are also mentioned by Kaśyapa[64] and Vāgbhaṭa,[65] which are responsible for inadequate milk secretion. These are—fear, travelling, hard labour, consumption of rūkṣa diet (having less calories due to less quantity of fat) and fasting.

Modern concept is quite similar to the Āyurvedic concept, because modern theory also considers that inhibition of milk secretion is mostly psychological in origin. It can be very acute; for examples sudden shock, a burst of anger, embarrassment or strong pain may result in what mother call 'drying up.' Possibly, the release of adrenaline in response to the stimulus, results in constriction of the blood vessels surrounding the alveoli, so that oxytocin does not reach the myoepithelial cells, so they do not contract. Instead, the alveoli relax, and the milk is no longer pushed forward.

Inhibition can also be more chronic. Continuous anxiety and worry inhibit both the let-down reflex and the milk-producing reflex.

Measures and Drugs for Increasing Milk Secretion (Stanya Janana Drugs)

Various recipes and measures have been mentioned in ancient texts, for increasing the production of breast milk. In Caraka Saṃhitā, following recipes have been mentioned:

1. All type of wines (except Sīdhu) are galactogouge.
2. Vegetables, cereals, flesh and milk of animals living in wildly or in marshy land or water.
3. Generally liquids and drugs (having madhura, amla and lavaṇa properties) and milk is beneficial for increasing milk secretion.
4. Use of decoction prepared with roots of Uśīra, Śāli, Śaṣṭika (both varieties of rice). Ikṣuvālikā, Darbha, Kuśa, Kāsa, Gundra, Itkaṭa, and Katṛṇa are beneficial.[66]

Suśruta opines that along with various recipes, psychology of mother also play an important role in increasing the milk secretion, and following measures are mentioned:

1. Dhātrī should keep herself cheerful.
2. Use of barley, wheat, rice (Sāthī and Śāli), meat-soup, wine, Kāñji, pasted Tila, Laśuna, fish, Kaseruka, Sṛngāṭaka, Bisa, Vidārīkanda, Madhuka, Śat āvarī, Nalikā, Alābu, Kālaśāka, etc.[67]

Kaśyapa[68] has given following recipes:

1. Vegetables (except śveta sarṣapa), meat-soup (except hog and buffalo), Garlic and Onion.
2. Decoction prepared with the bark of Vaṭādi and Kṣīrivṛkṣa cooked in milk and Pākyalavaṇa (Sauvarcala), Viḍa lavaṇa, ghṛta are added. This recipe should be taken with rice (śāli).
3. Milk medicated with decoction of rice (sāṭhī) and roots of Darbha, Kuśa, Itkaṭa, etc.
4. Nadikā (Kāla-śāka) cooked with jaggery and mixed with hingu and Jātiphala should be used with milk, meat-soup or wine.

Other texts[69] have also mentioned the above said drugs, however, Vāgbhaṭa has mentioned the drugs of 'Padmakādi gaṇa' which have property to enhance milk secretion.[70] This gaṇa includes following drugs Padmākha, Prapauṇḍarīka, Vṛddhi, Vaṃśalocana, Ṛddhi, Karkaṭaśrangī, Guḍūcī, drugs of Jīvanīya gaṇa (Jīvantī, Kākolī, Kṣīrakākolī, Medā, Mahāmedā, Mudgaparṇī, Māṣaparnī, Ṛsbhaka, Jīvaka and Madhuyaṣṭī.

Modern medicine still not have any satisfactory treatment for enhancing breast milk. Various prescriptions given by ancient scholars, may fulfil this deficiency.

REFERENCES

1. S.S.Sū. 35.34; K.S.Khil .3.72; A.H.U. 2.1
2. Vā.Pu. 31.23,24
3. C.S.Śā. 8.54
4. S.S.Sū. 45.49
5. K.S.Khil. 22. Kṣīraguṇa
6. H.S. 1.8.13
7. C.S.Śā. 8.54; C.S.Sū. 27.224
8. S.S. Ni. 10.26; S.S.Sū. 45.57
9. A.H.U. 1.15; Hā.S. 1.8.23; M.Bh. Śāntiparva.
10. Hā.S. 1.8.23
11. Hā.S. 1.8.13, 14
12. C.S.Ci. 15.17
13. S.S.Ni. 10.18 to 22; M.N. 67. 1-4
14. S.S.Ni. 10.23
15. K.S. Lehā.

16(a) K.S.Khil. 9.20, 21

16(b) K.S.Khil. 22

17. M.N. 67.1 to 4
18. Hā.S. 1.8.7 to 12
19. Hā.S. 1.8.7 to 10
20. Kumāra Sambhava
21. C.S.Śā. 8.54
22. S.S.Ni. 10.26
23. S.S.Śā. 10.35
24. K.S.Sū. 19
25. A.S.U. 1.21; A.H.U. 2.2; M.N. 68.4; G.N. 11.2
26. C.S.Śā. 8.52, 53
27. S.S.Śā. 10.28
28. S.S.Śā. 10.32
29. S.S.Śā. 10.36

30. K.S.Sū.Kṣiro
31. A.S.U. 1.20
32. A.S.U. 1.38
33. A.H.U.I. 15, 16
34. Divyā.II. 19; M.I. 395; II. 324; Jātaka I.57; III 391; Pr.A. 16. 176
35. Divyā.II. 19; Mahā Vagga I. 5.22
36. Mūgapakkha Jātaka XXII. 538
37. Kalpa Sū. 1.28 page 252; Bh. Sū. 4.11.11.29; Vi.Sū. 8 page 449
38. R.V.I. 164.49
39. C.S.Śā. 8.46
40. C.S.Śā. 8.58
41. S.S.Śā. 10.29 to 31
42. S.S.Śā. 10.33
43. A.S.U. 1, 22, 23
44. A.H.U. 1.20
45. S.S.Śā. 10.53; A.H.U. 1.20; C.D. 64.2; V.V. 69.2
46. C.S.Sū. 27.218
47. K.S.Khil. 22
48. A.H.Sū. 5.21 to 23
49. Hā. S. 1.8.15 to 18
50. C.S.Sū. 27.222
51. S.S.Sū. 45.68
52. K.S.Khil. 23
53. A.H.U. 5.24; Hā.S. 1.8. 19
54. S.S.Śā. 10.54. K.S.Khil. Jat. 12.15; A.H.U. 1.37
55. Pa.G.Sū.I. 19.4
56. Śā.G.S.I.27; Āp.G.S.I.16.1; Āsva. G.S.I.10, H.G.S.II.5
57. S.S.Śā. 10.54
58. K.S.Khil. Jāt. 12.15
59. A.H.U. 1.37 to 39

60. A.S.U. 1.43
61. K.S.Sū.Lehā.
62. C.S.Śā. 8.57
63. S.S.Śā. 10.34
64. K.S.Sū.Kṣīra. 19
65. A.S.U. 1.24; A.H.U. 1.17 to 18
66. C.S.Śā. 8.5; C.S.Sū. 4.17
67. S.S.Śā. 10.34
68. K.S.Sū.Kṣiro. 9.6 to 8
69. Y.R.S. 354 to 356; R.M.Strīroga. 38, 39; Hā.S. 457
70. A.H.Sū. 15.12

3

General Care of Children

The care of child is a very important aspect, related to their protection and maintenance of physical as well as psychological health. Various other aspects related to hygiene, cloths and toy also have their role in child health care. In ancient period, peoples were aware of these facts, therefore, ancient scholars have included their description in detail, which are discussed here, under following different headings.

1. Protective Measures

The immunological system of children is not fully developed, therefore, more susceptible for infections. Various measures have been adopted in ancient period for protection of children.

Suśruta opines that the children (especially infants) should be isolated and various external environmental contacts should be avoided to protect him from various infections including graha rogas.[1] Kaśyapa has prescribed certain 'lehas' which are supposed to enhance the non-specific immunity of children.[2] Similarly Karṇavedhana Saṃskāra.[3] described in various texts, may also provide active immunity due to trauma, apart from ornamental use.

Various measures used to protect the newborn (in Kumārāgāra) have been discussed previously in the Chapter 'Care of Newborn,' therefore, not included here. However, others are discussed as follows:

(a) *Use of Amulets*

Vedas advocate to wear Maṇis for prevention of diseases, increasing strength, destroying enemies, and for happy long life. Description of 9 types of Maṇis (amulets) are available in Vedic literature. These are Astrata, Audumbara, Jāngiḍa, Darbha, Pratisara, Phāla, Varaṇa, Ṣatvāra and Śaṃkha Maṇi. Except Śaṃkha Maṇi, others are vegetable products.[4]

Caraka opines that amulets made of various stones; horn of alive rhinoceros, deer, or nīlagāya (a kind of big white footed antelop); different herbal drugs like Andrī, Brāhmī, Jīvaka, Ṛsabhaka may protect the child from various evil powers and infections.[5] Vāgbhaṭa has also advocated these above articles as amulet. The amulet should be tied on wrist, neck or head.[6] In the book Rāja Mārtanda use of Mayūra śikhā is advocated for this purpose.[7]

The use of amulet, made by nails of Tiger (Vyāghra-nakha) was most prevalent in ancient period. Its frequent use is mentioned in the literature of Bāṇa. A sculpture of Kārtikeya (5th Century A.D.) has also found to have Vyāghra nakha (nails of tiger) amulet tied in the neck (Plate 2).

(b) *Fumigation (Dhūpana)*

Caraka,[8] Suśruta,[9] and Kaśyapa[10] have advised to perform fumigation of various articles (animal and vegetable origin) to protect from various infections, promotion of health and treatment of various disorders (especially graha). The detailed description will be discussed in description of Grahas, under the chapter "Diseases of Children."

(c) *Protection from poisons*

The newborn should be protected from the effects of various poisons, by administering them cow's ghṛta medicated with Kuṣṭha (Śweta) and honey. This concept in later period is mentioned by Harmekhalā.[11] Use of 'Viṣaghna mantra' is advocated in the book Rāja Māratanḍa.[12]

Scientifically, it is very difficult to explain the utility of amulets of mantras for proection, with the present available knowledge. However, conceptually, it can be explained as follows:

Mantras are composed of letters of the alphabet. Some mantras do carry a meaning but others are mostly meaningless, for a common man and they carry only secret tāntric implications. Whatever the meaning may or may not be, these mantras do not produce effects only because of the meaning they carry. Recitation of these mantras orally or mentally in a prescribed manner, creates a peculiar vibration in the individual. The energy thus produced, is transformed into the image or idol through the 'yantras' or even directly.

The objects like amulets, after sanctification and impregnation with the mantras, remain perpetually as a storehouse of energy, which can be acquired by the same or any other individual when needed for protection from various evil powers.

An other hypothetical explanation may also be given. During the ceremony and enchanting of Mantras a specific atmosphere is created. The whole atmosphere have its effect on the child already present there. The child follows the movements of hand, during recitation of mantras. It helps to concentrate the child. Mantras create a peculiar vibration which may produce electro-magnetic changes in the body and mind. Medicated smoke may also have its effect on child, after being inhaled. All these factors have their combined effect on child and may be responsible for changes in the body and ultimately initiating the defence mechanism.

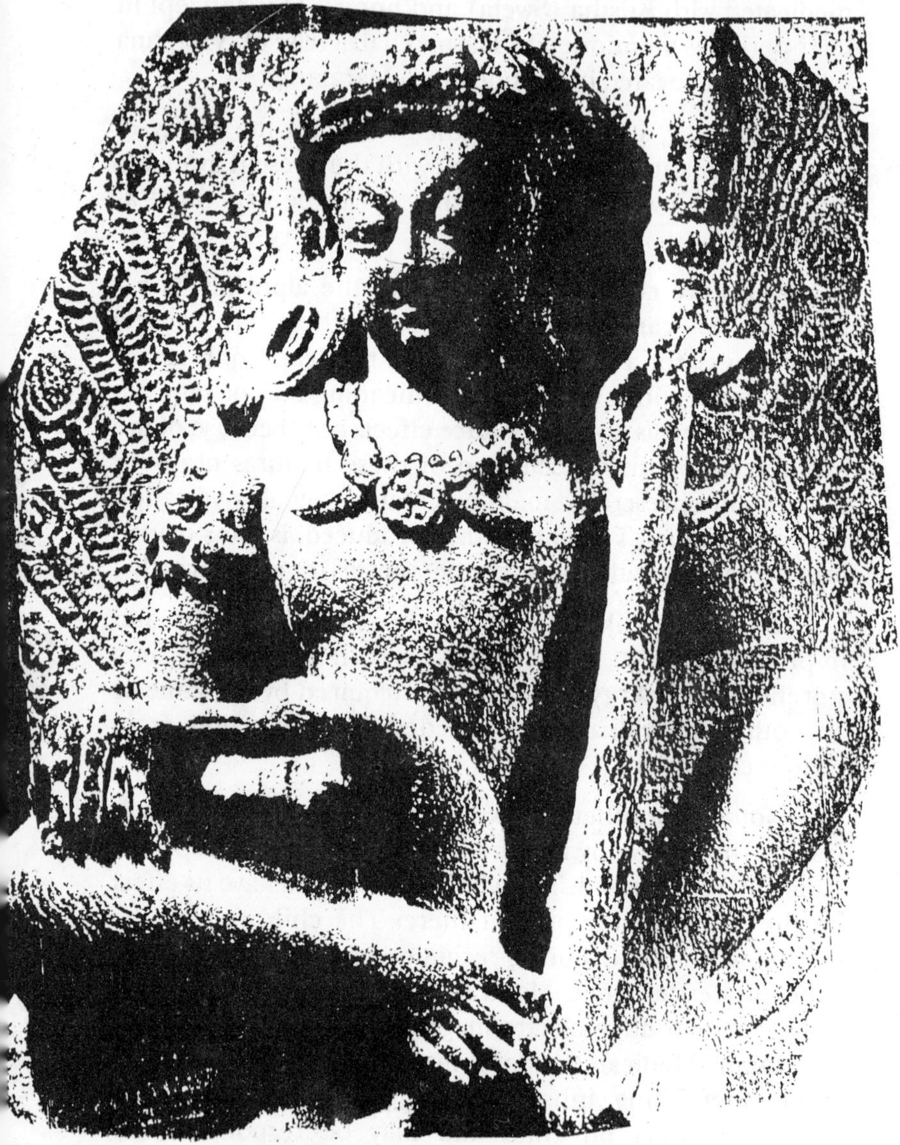

Plate 2—Sculpture of Kārtikeya (5th Century AD) Bearing amulet of tiger-nail (Vyāghra-nakha for protection from evil—demons (Courtesy: Bharat Kala Bhawan, B.H.U.)

2. General Care and Hygiene

General rules of hygiene and health care are very important because by observing these, one can keep his child healthy. Here references are recapitulated, which were prescribed by our ancient scholars.

(a) *Massage and anointments*

Caraka opines that massage is a effective procedure to provide strength to the skin.[13] Suśruta has advised to massage newborn with Balā-taila. Kaśyapa is of opinion that the child should be massaged during night. The child gets sound sleep due to its effect.[14] Vāgbhaṭa has described preparation of oil useful for massage and other anointments.[15]

Oil for massage—Oil medicated with Sahadevī, Śālaparṇī, Hareṇu, Kaunti, Kumuda, Utpala, Candana, Vṛhatī, Takkārī, Sarṣapa, Kuṣṭha, Saindhava, Aśvagandhā, Eraṇḍa-mūla, Tila, Apāmārga, Taṇḍul, fruits of Kauñca and goat's milk, should be used for massage.

Anointments—(i) The above drugs described for taila are mixed with cikkasa, curd and honey and used as anointment. (ii) Anointment made of Mūrvā-mūla, Haridrā, Dāruharidrā, and Yava. (iii) Anointment of Kulattha powder. (iv) Anointment made of Aśvagandhā Cūrṇa (powder).

In the book Rāja Mārtaṇḍa, Vacā and Baṭa-mūla are prescribed to prepare the oil for massage. The massage should be performed to the child exposing in sunlight. An anointment is also described in this book. It is prepared with the leaves of Saptacchada and Arka, roots of Naktamāla and Kanera with cow's urine. Application of it provides strength to child.[16]

Various drugs used for preparing the oil are absorbed through the skin and may have their systemic effect also. Massage in sunlight initiate the skin for synthesis of Vitamin D.

The act of rubbing the skin during massage provides strength and improves its blood supply. Thus, keeping it healthy and free from diseases along with psychological satisfaction of the child.

(b) ***Bath***

Caraka has described the benefit of bath. The body become clean and free from sweat and dust, by taking it properly.[17]

The water used for bath should be medicated with Kṣīri-Vṛkṣa-Kaṣāya or drugs of 'Sarvagandhodaka group' or with Kapitthpatra. These preparations are prescribed by Suśruta and Vagbhaṭa[18] while Rāja Mārtaṇḍa[19] has advised to give bath from water medicated with Hrībera and Muṇḍī or with Baṭa-mūla.

The bath with medicated water may provide aseptic care to the skin, maintenance of body heat along with systemic effect of the drugs, absorbed through skin.

(c) ***Cleaning of teeth***

It is the opinion of Vāgbhaṭa,[20] that brushing of teeth should be avoided in children uptill their gums are delicate. However, mouth wash from water should be done to clean his mouth.

(d) ***Use of water***

In Kaśyapa Saṃhitā,[21] use of drinking water for children is described as follows:

1. The child should be offered water, after completion of meal. If it is taken before or inbetween, the child may become weak.
2. Boiled and cooled water is very congenial to children and also effective in all disorders, except raktapitta.
3. The type of water should be selected according to the season.

Season	*Type of water*
1. Autumn (Śarada)	Rain water warmed in sunlight
2. Winter (Hemanta or Śiśira)	Water of pond and river
3. Summer (Grīṣma) and Spring (Vasanta)	Water of well and spring
4. Rainy season (Varṣā)	Boiled and cooled water or water of well.

Water prescribed during different season may be according to its availability. The boiled and cooled water, as described by Kaśyapa, is really good for children. On boiling the water become free from all bacteria. The Gastro-intestinal tract of children is very susceptible for any organism. The unboiled water may produce diarrhoea and other disorders. Thus use of boiled water prevents various water born diseases.

(e) ***Recipes congenial in different seasons***

Vāgbhaṭa[22] has mentioned the use of some recipes, which are congenial to children, in particular season. These may help in counteracting the effects of season.

(i) In Winter (Śita) and Spring (Vasanta)—Use of medicated ghṛta with decoction of drugs of Āragvadhādi group and paste of Vatskādi group of drugs.

(ii) In Summer (Grīṣma)—In the morning, use of cold milk medicated with drugs of Jīvanīya group, provide relief to the child from the effect of warm air, sun and sweating.

Use of ghṛta should be avoided, if child drinks much quantity of water. In case, where ghṛta is congenial then it should be given after medicating it with Kākolī, Medā, Vamśalocana, Madhuyaṣṭhī and Jīvaka.

Use of ghṛta medicated with drugs of Vidāryādi group, Rāsanā, Saralā, Punarnavā, Hingu, Saindhava, Devadāru.

(iii) In Autumn (Śarada)—Use of Kṣīra ghṛta medicated with Prapauṇḍarīka, Madhuyaṣṭhī, Mudgaparṇī, Māṣaparaṇī, Durālabhā, Priyāla majjā, Kākolī, Vidārī, Kaṭphala, Amṛtā, Drākṣā, Ajaṣrangī, Dugdhikā, Kṣīraśuklā, Aśvagandhā, Karkaṭa śrangī, flowers of Madhūka, Medā, Jīvaka and Ṛsabhaka.

(f) *Habit of pica*

Vāgbhaṭa has observed that some children might have habit of eating clay. The child may suffer from various disorders due to this bad habit. These disorders may be treated by offering ghṛta, medicated with Pāṭhā, Viḍanga, Haridrā, Dāruharidrā, Mustā, Bhārangī, Punarnavā, Bilva, Trikaṭu and Vṛścakālī.[23]

In modern literature, pica has been considered a habit disorder. It is most often associated with family disorganization, poor supervision, and affectional neglect. It appears to be more prevalent in lower socio-economic classes and may be related to poor nutrition. The treatment prescribed by Vāgbhaṭa supplies various nutrients along with medicaments, which may help to come up the problem.

3. Cloths and Bed

Caraka is of opinion that the bed, bedsheet and cloths, used for children, must be light, soft, clean, and fragrant. Dirty cloths should not be used and must be changed. These may be re-used only after proper washing, drying and fumigation.[24] Suśruta and Vāgbhaṭa[25] is also of similar opinion. This explains the high standard of hygiene practice during those days.

4. Handling of Baby

Children are very delicate, therefore, should be handled properly and carefully. Handling is not related upto physical care but it is also related with psychological care of the child. To perform this difficult job, the person, handling of child should also have few qualities.

(a) *Qualities of person handling the child (Kumārādhāra)*

Vāgbhaṭa has mentioned the qualities of person looking after the child. The person should be moral, religious, not too much obese and free from ambition.[26]

(b) *Handling*

Suśruta[27] has mentioned various points which should be considered, during handling of a child.

(i) The child should be handled very comfortably.

(ii) The child should not be allowed to sit for a long time, because it may develop deformities of vertebral column.

(iii) He/she should be protected from storm, strong sunlight, sparking during lightning, rain,.dust and smoke. These should be avoided very strictly upto the age of 1 year, as described by Vāgbhaṭa.

Vāgbhaṭa further opines that the child (especially infant) should be looked after during sleep that any cloth may not cover his mouth or nostrils. This may cause suffocation or even death.[28]

(c) *Psychological care*

Ancient scholars have given much stress on psychological care of children because during childhood period, the personality is in developing stage. Any psychological trauma may affect the whole personality.

The following points should be considered to take care of psychology of the child:

(i) The child should not be frightened.[29]

(ii) The child should not be tossed. On doing so the digestive system of the child may be disturbed, due to fear psychosis.[30]

(iii) He should not be left alone in dark or lonely places.[31]

Vāgbhaṭa has advised a recipe, which should be administered to children, to avoid fear psychosis. The recipe contains powder of Pippalī, Triphalā, ghṛta and honey.[32]

Fears are normal and perhaps a necessary part of psychologic development. The things which children are likely to fear that changes with age according to environment and experiences as they grow older. The younger child's fears are centred on basic conditions or situations such as darkness, or being left aone. Children may react immediately to traumatic events, or may keep their feelings dormant until maladaptive reactions become apparent during later periods of vulnerability. These facts were probably very well understood by ancient scholars, therefore, they have given too much stress on this aspect of child care.

5. Toys

Since the age of Sindhu civilization, hundreds of toys are acquired, which were used by children for their entertainments. In that civilization few common toys were—bull with moving head, monkey sliding on roap, whistle made of clay, figures of birds (Plate 3). As soon as the child could walk they used to pull along little carts or animals made of clay.

Such children's toys as have survived at Taxila (4th Century B.C.) are mainly of terra-cotta. That being the commonest and least destructible materials. These toys comprise:

(a) Toy carts drawn by a variety of animals—horse, bulls, rams and birds (Plate 3).

(b) Animals running on wheels (Plate 3).

(c) Animals without carts or wheels (Plate 4), and

(d) Rattles.

The Anguttarnikāya,[33] a Buddhist text has mentioned some toys to be played by the children. According to it a male child (kumāra), when he has grown older, plays with whatever may be the playthings of such children, such as a toy plough (vankaka), tip-cat (ghaṭikā), somersaults (mokkhacikā), wind mills (cingulaka), leaf-pannikins (paṭṭalhakam), toy-carts (rathakam) and toy bows (dhanukam). According to Jātaka literature, the boys used to make mountains of dust and girls play on filtering the sand. The famous play, Mṛcchakaṭikama also mentioned the use of toy-cart made of clay.

Mahābhārata has given description of flying of birds after tieing with thread. It was the favourite game of children, during those days.[34]

The poet Aśvaghoṣa has written that Gautama Buddha in his childhood was offered to play with toys—elephant, deer, horse, and bulls with charriot.[35] In Abhijñāna Śākuntalam, there is description of coloured peacock toys made of clay, which were used by Bharata to play. Playing with balls and dolls were the most favourite games of girls, in those days too.[36]

Toys of girls were different from those of boys. The Kāmasūtra has description of various games for girls, including making of garlands and small clay houses. A game played with stones was very popular in girls,[37] which is also played now-a-days too, by most of the village girls.

Āyurvedic texts, especially Caraka Saṃhitā, Kaśyapa Saṃhitā and Aṣṭānga Samgraha have given very illustrative description of toys and playgound.

Qualities of toys—The toys, given to children must have following qualities, as described by Caraka:[38]

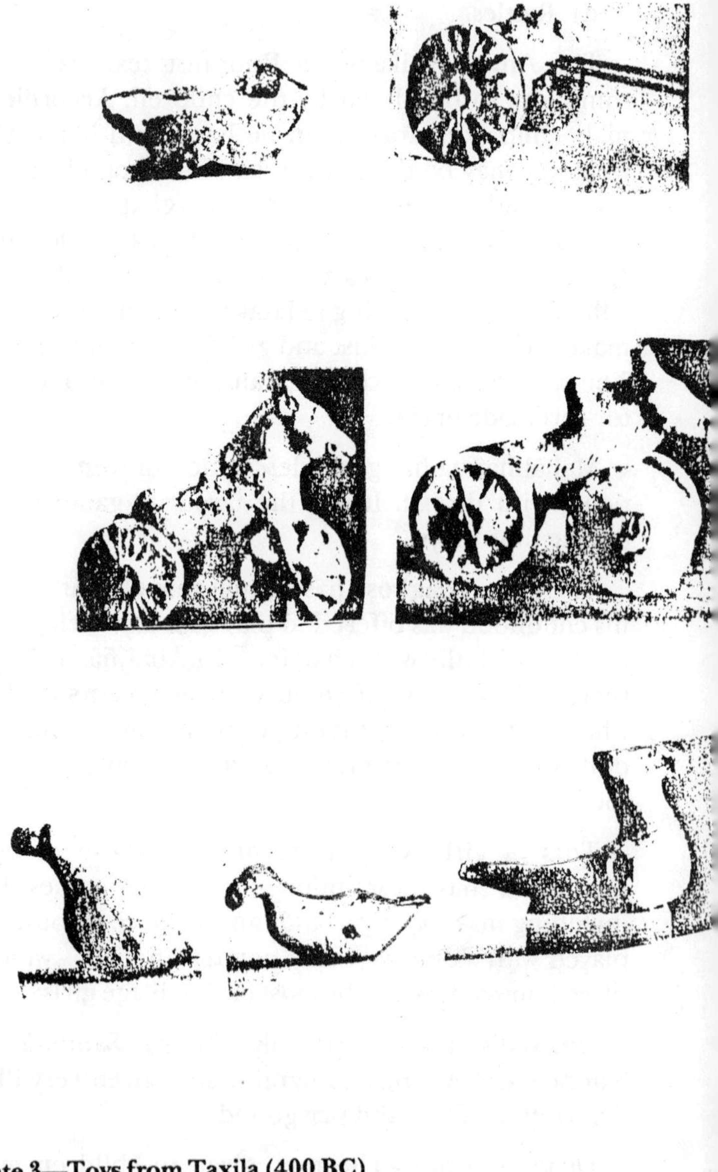

Plate 3—Toys from Taxila (400 BC)

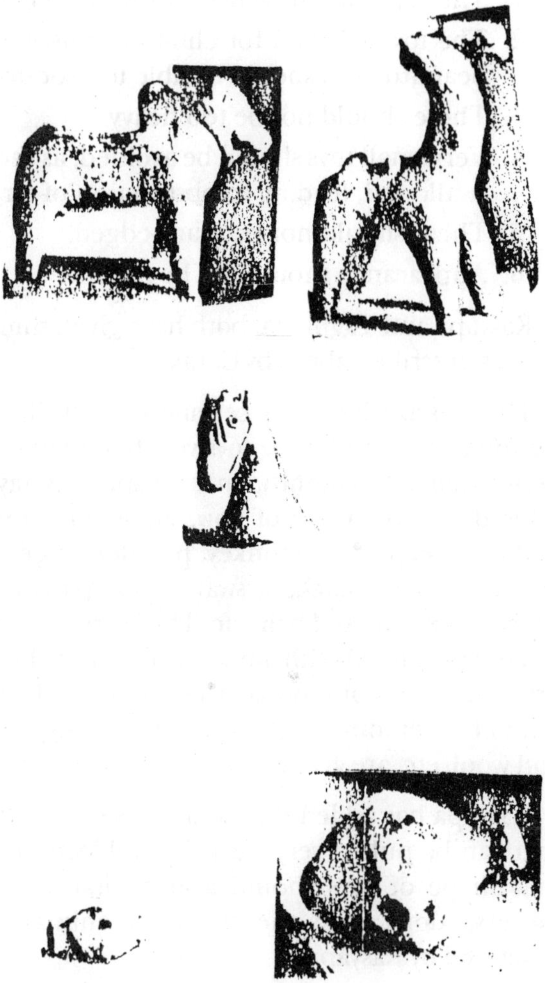

Plate 4—Toys from Taxila (400 BC)

1. The toys should be of different varieties.
2. The toys selected for children must be coloured and beautiful and should be able to produce sweet sound.
3. These should not be too heavy.
4. Very small toys should be avoided, as they can be easily swallowed, leading to obstruction of air passage.
5. These should not be sharp-edged.
6. Appearance should not be fearful.

Kaśyapa and Vāgbhaṭa, both have given similar qualities of toys, as described above by Caraka.[39]

The description of a ceremony is available in Kaśyapa Saṃhitā, for introducing toys very first time to the child. It is performed in 6th month, on an auspicious day. The toys first offered are in shapes of cow, elephant, camel, horse, ass, buffalo, sheep, goat, monkey, pig, deer, tiger, lion, tortoise, mainā (a bird), cuckoo, swan, cock, parrot, crane, house, chariot, boy, girl and ball, etc. These are prepared from flour of cereals, mixed with milk, curd, ghṛta, honey and cow's urine. The toys of food articles are offered only once at the time of ceremony, later on the toys made of wood, cotton and wool, etc. are given.[40]

Kaśyapa has added that some toys should be of such type that can be pulled very easily by children. Vābghaṭa opines that shape of toys should also be like that of fruits and flowers, along with the shape of animals, as previously described by Kaśyapa.

Playground—Vāgbhaṭa is the only scholar, who has considered the importance of playground for small children. He opines that the ground should be levelled and free from stones and other sharp and small objects, which may harm to children. The ground should be sprayed with water medicated with Viḍanga, Marica or Nimba.[41] These drugs are Kṛmighna, therefore, by this spray, the ground becomes free from insects, along with various protozoa and helminths. The child will also avoid to eat clay due to its bitter taste produced with the effect of drugs.

The above references regarding toys and playground indicate that the people of ancient period were aware of the importance of toys, and considered that toys are not for only entertainment of children but these also have their psychological impact. Modern texts of the subject are still behind and are not giving much importance to such an important aspect.

6. Education

Suśruta, Vāgbhaṭa and Kauṭilya have mentioned that the school education of a child must be started, as the child become able to receive it.[42]

The early school period of childhood starts from 6 years of age. By 5 years, the brain is fully developed and the child is ready for education and training.

7. Tonics for Children

In childhood period (especially in infancy), the rate of growth and development is very high. The preparations used as tonic for children may serve two purposes—to tone up the process of growth and development, and to provide supplementary nutrition. Texts of ancient period have mentioned several recipes to be used in children for the following purposes:

(i) To enhance growth and development by providing sufficient nutrients.

(ii) To enhance intelligence, and

(iii) For improving defective speech (delayed milestones).

Suśruta[43] has described four recipes (containing gold), which provide general immunity, body resistance and helpful in growth and development and enhancing the intelligence. These are:

(i) Svarṇa bhasma with Kuṣṭha, Vacā, Brāhmī, honey and ghṛta.

(ii) Svarṇa bhasma with paste of Brāhmī and Śankhapuṣpī should be given with honey and ghṛta.

(iii) Svarṇa bhasma, Arkpuṣpī, Vacā with ghṛta and honey.

(iv) Svarṇa bhasma, Kaiḍarya and Śveta Dūrvā with ghṛta.

Suśruta[44] has also mentioned few other general tonics for children of different age group:

(i) For breast fed babies (Kṣhīrāda)—Use of Vacā, Jaṭāmānsī, Apāmārga, Śatāvarī, Sārīvā, Brahmī, Pippalī, Haridrā, Kuṣṭha and Sanidhava with honey.

(ii) For breast fed and top fed (with cereals) babies (Kṣhīrānnāda)—Ghṛta medicated with Vacā, Madhuyaṣṭhī, Pippalī, Citraka and Triphalā.

(iii) For babies on full diet (Annāda)—Ghṛta medicated with Daśamūla, Tagara, Bhadradāru, Marica, Madhuyaṣṭhī, Drākṣhā and Brāhmī.

Kaśyapa[45] has named the preparations known as 'Leha.' The process by which these are introduced to the child is known as 'Lehana.'

Lehana

Indications of Lehana

(i) Children receiving inadequate amount of breast milk due to pregnancy of mother or any other reason.

(ii) Children having increased demand of food.

(iii) Children passing less amount of urine and stool.

(iv) For the children who are very lean and thin without any organic problem.

Contraindications

Lehana is contraindicated in the following conditions : The children of weak digestive power, sleepy, passing much amount of urine and stool, having small but strong body, and suffering from various disorders like diseases of head, āmaroga, fever, diarrhoea, jaundice, oedema, anaemia, cardiac problem, respiratory disorders, ano-rectal disorders, abdominal discomforts, flatulance, enlargement of thyroid, excessive vomiting and nausea.

Lehas

Lehas mentioned by Kaśyapa:

(i) Svarṇa Prāśana—Pure gold is rubbed in water on a clean stone and given with honey and ghṛta, to the newborn. This recipe promotes health, growth, complexion and strength (immunity).

It is very much effective for enhancing intelligence and its response can be achieved within a month, however, full response may be achieved by its continuous use for 6 months. Suśruta has also prescribed the above recipe, during the ceremony of 'Jāta Karma.'

(ii) Ghṛta medicated with Brāhmī, Maṇḍūkaparṇī, Triphalā, Citraka, Vacā, Śatapuṣpā, Śatāvarī, Dantī, Nāgabalā and Trivṛta.

Kaśyapa has prescribed to use 3 other medicated ghṛta for enhancing intelligence. These are—Pañcagavya ghṛta and Brāhmī ghṛta. The composition of these ghṛtas are not mentioned by Kaśyapa, but it is available in Caraka Saṃhitā.[46]

(iii) Ghṛta medicated with Mañjiṣṭhā, Triphalā, Brāhmī, Balā, Atibalā, and Citraka in an equal quantity should be licked with honey.

(iv) Ghṛta medicated with Kuṣṭha, Vaṭānkura, Sarṣapa (Pīta), Pippalī, Triphalā, Vacā and Saindhava is effective recipe for renovating the intelligence.

(v) Abhaya ghṛta—Ghṛta medicated with Brāhmī, Siddhārthaka, Vacā, Sārivā, Kuṣṭha, Pippalī, and

Saindhava. This ghṛta, along with his medhā-vardhaka activity, also protects from infestations of grahas.

(vi) Samvardhana ghṛta—Ghṛta medicated with Khadira, Praśniparṇī, Syandana, Saindhava, Balā, Atibalā, and Kebuka, is effective in children with delayed milestones.

(vii) Ghṛta medicated with Brāhmī juice, cow's or goat's milk, cow's ghṛta, Triphalā, Anśumatī, Drākṣhā, Vacā, Kuṣṭhā, Hareṇu, Pippalī, Pippalāmūla, Cavya, Citraka, Nāgara, Tvaka, Tejapatra, Bālaka, Uśīra, Śveta candana, Utpala, Padmaka, Śatavarī, Nāgabalā, Dantī, Pāṭhā, Priyangu, Devadāru, Haridrā, Dāruharidrā, Viḍanga, Guggulu, Jātipatra, drugs of Jīvanīya gaṇa and other drugs.

Vāgbhaṭa has also described few recipes, useful for promotion of health and enhancement of intelligence:

(i) The newborn baby should be offered paste of Andrī, Brahmī, Śankhapuṣpī, and Vacā with honey and ghṛta, in dose equivalent to hareṇu (a kind of pea) with the help of the leaf of Aśvattha (Pīpala).

(ii) Brāhmī, Balā, Anantā or Śatāvari any one of them is used to lick the child.[47]

(iii) Brāhmī ghṛta—Ghṛta medicated with Brāhmī, Sarṣapa, Vacā, Sārivā, Kuṣṭha, Saindhava and Pippalī. It is effective for physical as well as intellectual development.

Brahmī ghṛta has also mentioned by Kaśyapa, but he has not given its composition.

(iv) Sārasvata ghṛta—Ghṛta medicated in goat's milk, Harītaki, Trikṭu, Pāṭhā, Śigru, Saindhava and Vacā is useful for digestive power, intelligence, memory and speech.

(v) Infants should be prescribed Vacā and Svarṇa bhasma with honey and ghṛta. It protects from various infections along with improving intellect and speech.

(vi) Medicated ghṛta with Brāhmī, Harītakī, Pippalī, Kuṣṭha, Haridrā, Sārivā, Vacā, Jaṭāmansī, Kaiḍarya; is beneficial for infants.

In the above medicated ghṛta, Brāhmī can be replaced with other drugs, like—Dūrvā, Mūrvā, Brahma Sauvarcala, Laxmaṇā, Śveta Kaṇṭakārī, Avyanḍa, Śveta sarṣapa, Śatāvarī, Phalanī (Priyangu) ripened fruits of Brahatī and Rohiṣa.[48]

(vii) Aṣṭānga ghṛta—Ghṛta medicated with Vacā, Indulekhā, Manḍūkaparṇī, Śankhapuṣpī, Śatāvarī, Brahma Somā, Amṛta, Brāhmī and milk.[49]

(viii) Vacādi ghṛta—Ghṛta medicated with Vacā, Amṛtā, Śatī, Pathyā (Haritakī), Śankhinī, Viḍanga, Śuṇṭhī and Apāmārga. It is equally effective like Sārasvata Ghṛta.[50]

Śiśuklyāṇa ghṛta, mentioned by Vāgbhaṭa[51] is similar to Abhaya ghṛya as described by Kaśyapa. Vāgbhaṭa[52] has also included four recipes (containing gold) in his text, which are mentioned earlier by Suśruta.[53] Other texts like Kalyāṇa Kāraka, Gada Nigraha, Vangsena Samhitā, Hārīta Saṃhitā and Yogaratna Samuccaya have also described few recipes useful for enhancing health and intellect. Only in Gada Nigraha[54] some recipes are mentioned with different compositions. These are as follows:

(i) Ghṛta medicated with Kuṣṭha, Vacā, Harītakī, Brāhmī, and Svarṇa Kṣhīrī should be given with honey. It is useful for maintaining health.

(ii) Sweet-balls prepared with Piyāla, Madhuyaṣṭhī, Madhulājā, honey, sugar-candy and milk provides strength.

(iii) Ghṛta medicated with paste of Aśvagandhā and milk is of much nutritive value and provides strength.

(iv) The powder of Vacā, Madhuyaṣṭhī, Saindhava, Harītakī, Śuṇṭhī, Ajamoda, Kuṣṭha, Pippalī, and Jivaka used with honey and ghṛta, is effective in defective speech.

REFERENCES

1. S.S.Śā. 10.55
2. K.S.Sū.Lehā.
3. S.S.Śā. 16.1; S.S.Ci. 19.21
4. A.V. 19.31.46; 2.4; 19.28, 29, 30, 34, 35; 10.3,6; 4.6; 1.15, 35
5. C.S.Śā. 8.62
6. A.S.U. 1.37; A.H.U. 1.27
7. R.M.Bāla. 3
8. C.S.Śā. 8.61
9. S.S.U. 28.6; 29.7; 30.7; 31.7; 32.7; 34.6; 35.6; 37.7
10. K.S.Kalpa. Dhūpa.
11. H.M. 4. 339
12. R.M. Bāla. 16-17
13. C.S.Sū. 5.88-89
14. K.S.Ci., page 129
15. A.S.U. 1.62
16. R.M.Bāl. 12
17. C.S.Sū. 5.94
18. S.S.Śā. 10.13; A.S.U. 1.6
19. R.M.Bāl. 14
20. A.S.U. 1.75
21. K.S.Khil. 23
22. A.S.U. 1.64, 65
23. A.S.U. 2.96; A.H.U. 2.76
24. C.S.Śā. 8.60
25. A.S.U. 1.33
26. A.S.U. 1.57
27. S.S.Śā. 10.52
28. A.S.U. 1.59
29. C.S.Śā. 8.64; A.S.U. 1.59; A.H.U. 1.41
30. A.S.U. 1.3

31. S.S.Śā. 10.52
32. A.S.U. 2.84
33. Anguttanikāya
34. M.Bh. Virāṭa Parva 12.4
35. Buddha Carita 2.22
36. Kumārasambhava 1.29
37. Kāmasūtra of Vatsyāyana
38. C.S.Śā. 8.63
39. K.S.Jāt. 12.7, 8; A.S.U. 1.60
40. K.S.Jāt. 12.7, 8
41. A.S.U. 1.60
42. S.S.Śā. 10.57; A.S.U. 1.61; Kauṭ. Arth.
43. S.S.Śā. 10.72-74
44. S.S.Śā. 10.50
45. K.S.Sū. Lehā.
46. C.S.Ci. 9.36-41
47. A.S.U. 1.8
48. A.S.U. 1.69-73
49. A.H.U. 1.43, 44
50. A.H.U. 1.46
51. A.H.U. 1.42
52. A.H.U. 1.47, 48
53. S.S.Śā. 10.72-79
54. G.N. 11.60, 81

4

Dentition

Dentition is a natural phenomenon beginning from infancy and teeth play an important role in life. Atharva Veda has considered that if tooth first appears in upper jaw, it is inauspicious. To allay the bad effect of this, God should be prayed.[1] By this description, it is clear that in those days too, there was well observed concept of tooth eruption, that normally first temporary teeth erupts in lower jaw. Modern embryology and anatomy also consider that lower central incisor teeth appears first at the age of 6-9 months while upper incisors later at 8-10 months.

In Ayurvedic texts, Caraka and Suśruta have not given any specific description of dentition, however, Suśruta and Vāgbhaṭa have mentioned various disorders of teeth and gums like śītāda, dantapuppuṭa, dantaveṣṭa, dantavaidarbha, vardhana, adhimānsa, dantanāḍī, dantavidradhi, krimidanta, dantaharṣa, bhanjanaka, danta śarkarā, kapālikā, caladanta, etc. Mādhava Nidāna has described the features of eight diseases of teeth. All these diseases are not specific for childhood period, but may affect the person of any age group, therefore, not described here.

Kaśyapa is the pioneer in this field. Different aspects of dentition are dealt in Kaśyapa Saṃhitā in a separate chapter

"Dantajanmikā." In this chapter, there is list of questions regarding dentition, which are raised by Jīvaka and explained by Kaśyapa. Though this chapter is incomplete due to missing portion of manuscript, therefore, it does not provide complete information of the subject. However, available description is informative and gives important clues of subject available in ancient period. Kaśyapa has following concept regarding dentition:[2]

1. Total teeth are 32 in number, out of which eight are 'Sakṛjjāta' (appear only once in life and remain in same form) and remaining are 'dvija.'
2. Milk (deciduous teeth) erupt in the same month, corresponding the month of intra-uterine life in which the formation of teeth begin.

   The month in which the child cuts its teeth, corresponds to the year in which temporary fall and permanent teeth begin to grow.
3. Names of various teeth have been given by Kaśyapa. These are: Rājadanta, Vasta, Daṃṣṭrā and Hānavya.

   The middle two teeth are Rājadanta (incisors) and are considered sacred. If these are broken, the person was considered unworthy for religious act. Teeth by the side of Rājadanta are called Vasta (Canines) and other teeth by the side of it are called Daṃṣṭrā (pre-molar). The rest are called Hānavya (molars) and named because are helpful in mastication.
4. Teeth erupt earlier in female than male, because their teeth are distant and soft, while stronger in male. Girls feel less problem than boys during teeth eruption.
5. Formation, eruption, growth and development, fall, their strength and weakness all depend on certain factors like—race, nature, maternal and paternal factors (hereditary) and acts of past life.

Vāgbhaṭa's notion regarding eruption and fall of tooth is similar to Kaśyapa. He also opines that cutting of teeth starts usually before the age of 8 months.[3]

Time of eruption and shedding of the primary teeth and eruption of permanent teeth, as accepted by modern anatomists and dentists is mentioned in the Table 2 and 3.

Table 2: Time of eruption and shedding of the primary teeth

	Eruption		*Sheddings*	
	Lower	*Upper*	*Lower*	*Upper*
	(Age in months)		*(Age in years)*	
1. Central incisor	6	$7\frac{1}{2}$	6	$7\frac{1}{2}$
2. Lateral incisor	7	9	7	8
3. Cuspid	16	18	$9\frac{1}{2}$	$11\frac{1}{2}$
4. First molar	12	14	10	$10\frac{1}{2}$
5. Second molar	20	24	11	$10\frac{1}{2}$

(From Massler and Schour; Atlas of the mouth. Chicago, American Dental Association).

Table 3: Time of eruption of the permanent teeth

		Lower *(Age in years)*	*Upper* *(Age in years)*
1.	Central incisors	6-7	7-8
2.	Lateral incisors	7-8	8-9
3.	Cuspids	9-10	11-12
4.	First bicuspids	10-12	10-11
5.	Second bicuspids	11-12	10-12
6.	First molars	6-7	6-7
7.	Second molars	11-13	12-13
8.	Third molars	17-21	17-21

Formation and Eruption of Teeth

By observing the last incomplete stanza of 'Dantajanmikā' chapter (Kaśyapa Saṃhitā), it can be presumed that this stanza might have had a detailed description of the process of tooth formation. In the last line of this stanza, there is clue regarding the description related to origin of teeth. According to it, during intra-uterine life, some amount of blood is collected in the pits of teeth. This blood by further development take the shape of teeth.[4]

In the text Aṣṭānga Samgraha, Vāgbhaṭa opines that tooth originates basically from Majjā and Asthi. Primary or milk teeth are weak and fall due to immature dhātus, but the secondary or permanent teeth are hard and strong since, they are made of mature dhātus.

The teeth do not appear again, if broken down by an injury or fallen due to any disease. Vāgbhaṭa has given very reasonable answer to it and explained that by the injury, the dhātubīja (germ), responsible for the development of teeth; are destroyed. The nutrition of teeth is also hampered due to injury of blood vessels. The dhātubīja (germs) and blood vessels can not be reoriginate, hence, development of teeth is affected.[5]

The concept of Vāgbhaṭa regarding genesis of teeth is more nearer to the facts. He opines that dhātubīja is basically responsible for further development of tooth. Dhātu-bīja can be very well considered as tooth buds, localized proliferations of cells in the dental laminae. These buds, which grow into the mesenchyme, develop into the deciduous teeth. The first indications of development appear early in the 6th week. The tooth buds for the permanent teeth with deciduous predecessors begin to appear at about ten fetal weeks, from continuation of the dental lamina, and they lie lingual to the deciduous tooth buds. The permanent molars which have no deciduous predecessors develop as buds from backward extension of the dental lamina. Tooth development is a continuous process, but it is usually divided into stages—bud, cap and bell stage.

Anodentia (Absence or Agenesis of Teeth)

Vāgbhaṭa has mentioned the physio-pathology of agenesis of teeth. He opines that the vāyu, situated in gums gets vitiated, either itself or with the help of pitta, dries up Asthi and Majjā. Because Asthi and Majjā are chief components of teeth, therefore, by drying these, there is no eruption of teeth.[6] Vangasena has considered that only vāyu is responsible for drying the gums (dantaveṣṭa) and ultimately for agenesis of teeth. Seat of this vāyu is root of teeth.[7]

By drying bīja of dhātus (asthi and majjā), there is absence of tooth buds. Total anodentia often occurs with ectodermal dysplasia. Partial anodentia results when a normal site of initiation is disturbed, as in the area of palatal cleft, or form genetic failure to code of the formation of specific teeth. The third molars, maxillary lateral incisors, and mandibular second premolars are the teeth that most commonly fail to form.

Types of Dentition

Kaśyapa has mentioned four types of dentition:[8]

1. Sāmudga,
2. Saṃvṛta,
3. Vivṛta, and
4. Danta sampata.

1. Sāmudga—Sāmudga means a joint with a socket, like a cup. This types of teeth develop in the condition of kṣaya (malnutrition) of child. These teeth use to fall very frequently.

2. Saṃvṛta—These are inauspicious and remain dirty.
3. Vivṛta—This type of teeth, causes excessive salivation. Because these are not fully covered with lips, there are much chances of diseases of teeth.
4. Danta Sampata—These are auspicious teeth having all the characteristics of healthy teeth.

Time of eruption of teeth and its effect

It has been observed by Kaśyapa that if eruption of teeth takes place before the age of 8th month, there are always chances of complications in teeth. Complication of teeth appeared in different months, are as follows[9] in Table 4.

Table 4: Period of teeth eruption and their effects

Period	*Effect*
4th month	Weak, fall very easily and diseased
5th month	Loose and diseased
6th month	Defective in shape, dirty, discoloured and affected with caries
7th month	Cracked having lines, broken, dry and forwardly protruded
8th month	Have all the qualities of a healthy tooth.

Vāgbhaṭa is also of similar views and opines that 8th month is appropriate for eruption of teeth in a healthy child. Children in which teeth erupt before the age of 8th months, should be considered having short and medium life span. He has pointed out an another fact that early eruption of teeth, due to excessive pain, causes defective maturation of dhātu-bīja.[10]

Vangasena has different concepts regarding the effects of early dentition. According to him, family members of the child are affected, if dentition occur before the age of 8th month. The child who has dentition in one, two or three months of age, is inauspicious for his father, brother, mother, parents, and all the family members including servant and teacher, etc. if dentition takes place in fourth, fifth, sixth and seventh months respectively.[11]

There is no any specific cause of premature eruption of teeth which is mentioned in modern literature. However, few have considered that endocrine factors may be involved because premature eruption of teeth sometimes occurs in infants with congenital adrenal hyperplasia. Concepts of ancient scholars have favoured this cause of premature eruption of teeth, which is clear from following points:

1. Vāgbhaṭa has considered that children having very early eruption of teeth have short and medium life span. Congenital adrenal hyperplasia may attribute four syndroms—Adrenogenital syndrome, cushing syndrome, hyperaldrosteronism and feminization. Children suffering from these disorders may have short life span.
2. Vangasena are more nearer to modern view point because he believes that due to early dentition of the child his family members are affected. If the cause of early dentition is considered congenital adrenal hyperplasia, then the claim of Vangasena becomes true since this defect is inherited as an autosomal recessive trait, therefore, can affect other family members.

Infant Born with Teeth (Sadanta Śiśu)

Sadanta Śiśu means a child born with teeth. In ancient period, such children were considered inauspicious. Vāgbhaṭa has described that in Sadanta Śiśu, if erupted tooth is in upper jaw, it is inauspicious.[12] Probably this concept has come from Vedas.[13]

In Aṣṭānga Saṃgraha, Vāgbhaṭa has mentioned a procedure to pass off the bad effect of a child born with teeth. For this purpose Lājā and honey is filled in the mouth of calf and his face is turned towards east. Now child is said to kiss the mouth of calf, three times. Besides this the child is carried on a boat or elephant, after giving a proper bath. Pāyasa (rice cooked in milk and mixed with honey and ghṛta) should be offered to Brāhmins.[14] Naigmeṣa graha is also worshipped for this purpose.[15] Soḍala has followed this procedure.[16] However, Vangasena has certain difference of opinion and considered that this type of children are very dangerous like demon because they kill their mother very shortly.[17]

Modern literature consider that presence of teeth at birth, may be part of the normal dentition. These teeth are termed as 'Natal teeth' and observed in approximately 1 in 2000 newborn infants, usually there are 2 in the position of the mandibular central incisors. Their attachment is generally limited to the gingival margin, with little root formation or bony support. Such teech should not be considered supernumerary unless this is established roentgenographically. A natal teeth may be prematurely erupted primary teeth which suggests that early dental eruption may be expected. Vangasena is very right in his view that the infants having natal teeth is very dangerous to the mother, because they may produce maternal discomfort due to the abrasion or bitting of the nipple during feeding. Presence of natal teeth may also be due to congenital syphilis. Mother suffering from syphilis may transmit her disease to his baby developing in her womb.

Methods Helping Easy Dentition

Vāgbhaṭa, in the text Aṣṭānga Hṛdaya, has mentioned the following recipes for easy and painless eruption of teeth:

1. Powder of Pipplī or Dhātakī puṣpa and Āmalaki fruits with honey should be rubbed on gums, for easy dentition.
2. Application of dry flesh (māṃsa) of certain birds like Baṭera (Pheasant) and Tittar (Partridge) with honey helps appearance of teeth and mouth appears with teeth like lotus with pollen.
3. Use of Ghṛta medicated with Vacā, Bṛhatī (both), Pāthā, Kuṭakī, Atīsa, Mothā and drugs of Jīvanīya gaṇa.[18]

Rāja Mārtaṇḍa has advised a recipe for this purpose. Powdered dry flesh of Kuraka and Kapiñjala birds mixed with honey should be offered to the child.[19]

Texts of later period like Yogaratna Samuccaya.[20] Gada Nigrha[21] and Vangasena[22] have mentioned similar recipes, as mentioned by Vāgbhaṭa.

Qualities of Healthy Teeth and Gums (Praśasta Danta and Dantabandhana)

Kaśyapa has mentioned that healthy teeth should be properly developed, equal, strong, soft, smooth, pure, free from ailments, milky white in colour and well shaped.

The term 'dantabandhana' has been used for gums, by Kaśyapa. Healthy gums should be slightly elevated, red, soft, slightly hard and strong.[23]

Features of Defective Teeth (Apraśasta Danta)

Kaśyapa, while describing the dentition at 4th month, has mentioned the features of defective dentition and teeth. The main features are—appearance of teeth in intra-uterine life, scattered, less or more in number, very large, discoloured and broad shaped.[24]

Like Kaśyapa Saṃhitā, modern texts have also mentioned various abnormalities of teeth:

1. Enamel Hypoplasia—Defective enamel formation results in grooves, pits or fissures on the enamel surface. These conditions result from a temporary disturbances in enamel formation. Various factors may injure the amelblasts (e.g. nutritional deficiency, tetracycline therapy, diseases such as measles, and ingestion of high levels of chemicals such as fluoride). Rickets during the critical period of permanent tooth development is the most common known cause of enamel hypoplasia.
2. Abnormalities in shape—Abnormally shaped teeth are relatively common. Occasionally spherical masses of enamel, called enamel pearls (or drops), are attached to the tooth.
3. Numerical Abnormalities—One or more supernumerary teeth may develop.
4. Fused Teeth—Occasionally a tooth bud divides or two buds partially fuse to form fused or jointed teeth. In some cases the permanent tooth does not form; this suggests that the deciduous and permanent tooth primordia may have fused.
5. Amelogenesis inperfecta—The enamel is soft and friable because of hypocalcification, and the teeth are yellow to brown in colour.

Disorders of Dentition

Vāgbhaṭa and other scholars of later period have considered that during dentition, the child may suffer from various disorders like fever, headache, thirst, vertigo, diseases of eyes like Kukūṇaka and Pothaki, vomiting, cough, respiratory troubles, diarrhoea and skin disorders like Visarpa.[25]

Pathogenesis: Although various scholars have mentioned about disorders of dentition, however, Vāgbhaṭa has given its elaborate definition. Asthi and Majjā dhātus on maturation reach to Dantāśaya and produce some irritation. The child feel itching sensation on gums (due to Kapha situated in gums) so, he may bite the breast during sucking. Whatever article, the child finds, bites and presses it with gums to relieve itching pain. Vitiated vāyu, in association of Kapha reaches to asthi and majjā and spreads in whole body. At the same time, vāyu itself or with the help of pitta, vitiates other dhātus and malas and produces various complications during dentition.[26]

Further, he has compared vitiated doṣas (at the time of dentition) with the example of cat and peacocks, and opines that in children, at the time of dentition all the doṣas, dhātus and even malas are vitiated like vitiation occurring in cats after breaking of their vertebral column (Pṛṣṭha bhanga) or during growth of feathers in Peacock.[27] Soḍala, in his text Gada Nigraha, has also given similar example.[28]

As the teeth penetrate the gums, inflammation and sensitivity sometimes occur, a condition referred to as teething. The child may become irritable and salivation may increase markedly. Bacterial invasion through a break in the tissue or under a gingival flap, covering the teeth, may be responsible. A blunt, firm object for the infant to bite usually provides some relief; incision of the gums is seldom indicated. There is no definite evidence to support claims of accompanying temporary systemic disturbances, such as low-grade fever, facial rashes and mild diarrhoea. However, there may be one possibility that during dentition, due to irritation of gums, children use to bite any object they find. These objects may be dirty and possibly can transfer various micro-organisms, responsible for respiratory, gastro-intestinal and other disorders.

Treatment

Vāgbhaṭa and Cakrapāṇi (Cakradatta) have advised not to treat disorders of dentition, because these subside in due course, as the dentition completes.[29] But at the same time beside this opinion, they have mentioned treatment of disorders also. By this it can be inferred that disorders associated with dentition should be over looked, if mild, but a proper treatment is necessary for moderate or severe symptoms.

General treatment: Following recipes have been mentioned in different texts, for general management of dentitional disorders:

Ghṛta medicated with decoction of Mañjiṣṭhā, Dhātakī puṣpa, Lodhra, Kuṭannaṭa (Śyonāka), Balā, Atibalā, Mahāsahā (Śālparṇī), Kṣudrasahā (Māṣaparṇī), Mudgaparṇī, Bilva (Unripped), fruits of Kārpāsa, relieves all general complaints of dentition.[30]

Vāgbhaṭa, after describing this recipe, mentioned that this recipe is described by Vṛddha Kaśyapa, however, in Kaśyapa Saṃhitā there is no description of this recipe. Therefore, it may be possible that Kaśyapa Saṃhitā, available during the period of Vāgbhaṭa might be containing that recipe, which has been missed later on in present available Kaśyapa Saṃhitā.

This recipe is also mentioned in Aṣṭānga Hṛdaya and Gada Nigraha.[31]

The book Hermekhalā has description of two recipes for general management of dentitional disorders:

1. Roots of Sitasinduvāra, collected from east side should be tied in the neck of the child. It may prevent various disorders associated with dentition.
2. Roots of Dugdhalikā, Śankhapuṣpī, Tumbī, Yavāsā should be tied in the neck for above purpose.[32]

Bhoja, the writer or Rāja Mārtaṇḍa[93] has followed Hermekhalā.

Treatment of Individual Ailments During Dentition

It is only Vāgbhaṭa,[94] who has mentioned detailed description, in his text Aṣṭānga Saṃgraha, regarding management of different disorders appearing during dentition.

1. *Treatment of fever*

(a) Decoction made with Devadāru, Mustā, Madhuyaṣṭhī, Mañjiṣṭhā and sugar-candy cures vātika fever.

(b) Decoction of Bhadradāru, Mustā, Madhuyaṣṭhī, Vidārī, Śālaparṇī, Praśnaparṇī and Śatāvarī or Ghṛta medicated with these drugs cure Vātika jvara (fever). This ghṛta may also be used for massage.

(c) Oil medicated with Haridrā, Kuṣṭha, Vacā, Śatpuṣpā, Hareṇu, Bhārangī, Elā, Susavī (Kalaunjī), Rāsanā, Punarnavā, Tagara and Sarṣapa should be used for massage.

2. *Treatment of diarrhoea, thirst and vomiting*

(a) Pittaja jvara and Atisāra may be cured by the use of powder of Lājā, Nīlakamala, Pippalī, Yaṣṭī, Añjana and Śarkarā (sugar) with honey.

(b) Use of decoction of Lājā, Pippalī, Gajapippalī with śarkarā (sugar) and honey, will cure jvara (fever), atisāra (diarrhoea), thirst and vomiting.

(c) To get relief from Āmātisāra (diarrhoea with mucus) or Raktātisāra (diarrhoea with blood), the powder of Gajapippalī with sugar or powder of Devadāru with sugar should be used.

(d) Thirst may be relieved by giving boiled and cooled water, medicated with the powder of Mavādanī (Indrāyaṇa) and Dāḍima.

(e) Powder of Priyangu, Rasāñjana and Mustā with water of rice and honey is used to get relief from thirst, diarrhoea and vomiting.

3. *Headache*

(a) Anointment of cold ghṛta relieves headache.

(b) Paste of leaves of Kapittha, Cāngerī, Plum and Kākamācī, applied to forehead cures headache, vomiting and diarrhoea.

4. *Complications of Eye*

Kukūṇaka and Pothakī diseases should be treated separately, Vāgbhaṭa has mentioned only general management of complications of eyes, appearing during dentition.

Application (in eyes) of a wick prepared with the pieces of Piappalī, Muñja, buds of Jasmine, Barley and leaves of Nīlakamala (each 100 in number), cures general complications of eye.

5. *Fever, Diarrhoea, Cough, Anemia (Paṇḍu) and disorders caused by mother (Mātrajanya doṣa)*

Powder of Paṭola, Nimba, Kuṭaja, Saptaparṇī, Ajamoda, Devadāru, Viḍanga, Sarala kāṣṭha with honey and ghṛta, is used to cure fever, diarrhoea, cough, anemia and disorders caused by mother.

6. *Fever (Kaphaja) and Skin disorder (Visarpa)*

The massage of oil made with the Śobhāñjana, paste made of Rāsanā, Elā, Tagara, Agnimantha (Sweet), Devadāru, Bilva, Kuṣṭha, Varaṇā, Hareṇu, Śatpuṣpā; cures fever.

Rounded eruptions, appearing due to vitiation of Kapha, can be cured by application of ghṛta, mixed with urine of elephant.

Diet During Dentition

For better dentition, Vāgbhaṭa has prescribed that the child should be provided milk and other laghu and bramhaṇa diet. Milk should not be discontinued suddenly from the diet of children.[35]

Milk is the best source of calcium. The requirement of calcium is increased during dentition. Thus, the milk can fulfil this requirement of calcium.

With the available ancient references about dentition, it is clear that Kaśyapa Saṃhitā is the text which contains the description of various aspects of dentition. Its description is nearer to the knowledge of todays accepted by modern literature. Vāgbhaṭa has tried to emphasize some aspects of the subject, like, development of teeth, pathogenesis and management of various ailments appearing during dentition. Vangasena has also given very few ideas, however, contribution of other ancient scholars in the subject is nominal.

REFERENCES

1. A.V.6. 13.140. 1 to 3
2. K.S.Sū.Dant. 20.4 to 5
3. A.S.U. 2.45
4. K.S.Sū. Dant. 20.34th page of Tāḍa Patra.
5. A.S.U. 2.21 to 27
6. A.S.U. 2.24
7. V.S.Bāl. 136
8. K.S.Sū. Dant. 20.7
9. K.S.Sū. Dant. 20.34th page of Tāḍa Patra
10. A.S.U. 2.20
11. V.S.Bālaroga. 140 to 148
12. A.S. 2.62; A.H. 2.62; B.S.Bāl. 140
13. A.V. 6.13.140.1 to 3
14. A.S.U. 2.63
15. A.S.U. 2.62
16. G.N. 11.116 to 118
17. V.S.Bāl. 140
18. A.H.U. 2.35 to 37
19. R.M.Bāla roga. 7
20. Y.R.S. 21.411
21. G.N. 11.33 to 35, 95
22. V.S.Bāla. 137, 138
23. K.S.Sū. Dant. 20. 34th page of Tāḍa Patra.
24. K.S.Sū. Dant. 20.6
25. A.S.U. 2.19; A.H.U. 2.26, 27; Y.R.S. 21.408,409; G.N. 11.24
26. A.S.U. 2.23
27. A.S.U. 2.24; A.H.U. 2.28
28. G.N. 11.25
29. A.S.U. 2.44; A.H.U. 2.43; C.D.Bāla. 52
30. A.S.U. 2.43

31. A.H.U. 2.42; G.N. 11.36, 37
32. H.M. 4.343, 344
33. R.M.Bāla. 5, 6
34. A.S.U. 2.32 to 38, 40
35. A.H.U. 1.37

5

Childhood Saṃskāras

The word 'Saṃskāra' is derived from the root 'Kri' with 'sam' upasarga (prefix), which is used for several meanings according to reference to context. Mīmaṃsakas consider it a ceremony for purification of sacrificial material, whereas Jaiminī Sūtras used it in the sense of some purificatory rite.[1] The commentator of Jaiminī Sūtras[2] has termed Saṃskāras as a purpose. According to Tantravārtika, the word 'Saṃskāra' can be considered as those arts and rites that impart fitness. The Naiyāyikas used it in the sense of producing self-reproductive quality and faculty of impression.

In the classical Saṃskrit texts, the word 'Saṃskāra' is used in a very wide sense, viz. in the sense of education,[3] cultivation, training,[4] refinement, polishing, embelishment, decoration and ornament,[5] a purificatory rite or ceremony to change the qualities.[6]

In short, the word 'Saṃskāra' means those religious rites and ceremonies which sanctify the body, mind and intellect so that the person may become fit for the society.

In other words, 'Saṃskāra' means 'guḍāntarādhāna' which is used for transform the qualities. Physicians can also assess the proper growth and development of child, during performing the saṃskāras.

Saṃskāras are the main field of Gṛhya Sūtras. In different Gṛhya Sūtras the number of Saṃskāras are different and vary from 12 to 18. Gautama Dharma Sūtra has a list of 40 Saṃskāras, while Manu Smṛti counted these 13 in numbers. These Saṃskāras are performed from conception till death. At present 16 Saṃskāras are in practice.

The present topic is related to children, therefore, various Saṃskāras performed, during childhood are mentioned here with their medical interpretations.

1. Jātakarma (Ceremony Performed After Birth)

The world 'Janman' or 'birth' has come several times in Ṛg Veda.[7] In Atharva Veda, there is a full hymn containing prayer and spells for easy and safe delivery.[8] In the Gṛhya Sūtras this Saṃskāra is described in detail. The Dharma Sūtras and the Smṛtis do not give detailed description.

According to Gṛhya Sūtras, the Jātakarma ceremony has performed before the cutting of the Umbilical Cord but the Caraka has described to perfrom it just after cutting of Umbilical Cord. After delivery of the child this good news was brought to the father. The cherished desire for a son as he freed the father from all ancestral debts. After this mother of the child is allowed to see the face of the son and then Jātakarma ceremony is performed. This ceremony has following socio-medical importance:

(a) *Medhā Jnana* (Promotion of intellect)—It is the main object of this Saṃskāra.[9] For this purpose the father with his fore-fingers and instrument of gold, gives honey and ghṛta or ghṛta alone to the child. Caraka described, Ghṛta is a beneficial substance for memory, intellect and talent.[10] The properties of honey and gold are equally favourable to the mental progress of the child.

Honey and ghṛta are rich source of carbohydrate and fat, respectively. These may provide energy to the child, even used in small quantity.

(b) *Āyuṣya* (for longevity)—It may be the purpose of this Saṃskāra. It is for ensuring a long healthy and happy life for the child.

According to Pāraskara Gṛhya Sūtra, the father does chanting of mantras near right ear of the newborn—'Agni is long lived; through the herbs etc. The Brāhman is long lived, through amṛtatwa, etc. The Rishis are long lived through observance, etc.; Sacrifice is long lived through sacrificial fire, etc.; The ocean is long lived through the rivers, etc.'[11]

An another method is also described for prolonging the life of the child. Father should invite five Brāhmans. They should sit towards five regions and should breath upon the child. One in the south with "back-breathing;" one to the west, "down-breathing," one to the north, "out-breathing" and fifth looking upwards "on-breathing."[12] The breathing was thought to be productive of life, therefore, this ceremony was performed to strengthen the breath of the child and prolong the life of child.

(c) *Strength*—Next purpose of Jātakarma Saṃskāra is to provide strength to the new born. The father perform this rite. He ask the new born, "Be a stone, be an ox, be an imperishable gold. Thou indeed art the self called son; thus live a hundred autumns."[13] In this saṃskāra during the process of giving honey and ghṛta to the newborn, the attending physician may observe for rooting, sucking and swollowing reflexes of newborn. Rooting reflex appears with birth and normally disappears upto the age of 9 months. It enables him to find the breast or finger having honey and ghṛta, without being directed to it. Its absence since birth to

9 months indicate bulbar palsy and hypotonia. Similarly sucking reflex is present since birth and disappears by 4th month (awake) and 7th month (asleep). Its absence in the stipulated period indicate that the newborn is depressed, sick or premature. If these reflexes are absent and feed is given forcefully then it may cause aspiration of food material (milk, honey, etc.) which may prove fatal.

2. Nāmakaraṇa (Naming Ceremony)

With the evaluation of language, men have tried to give names to things which are in daily use of their life. Men themselves were also named with the progress of social consciousness. The word 'Nāman' is found in Ṛg Veda.[14] The Ṛg Veda recognizes a secret name and the Aitareya[15] and Śatapatha Brāhmana,[16] refer to it.

In Gṛhya Sūtras there is detailed description about the composition of the name. According to the Pāraskara Gṛhya Sūtra,[17] the name should be of two syllables or of four syllables, beginning with asanant, with a semi-vowel in it, with the long vowel or the Visarga at its end, with a kṛt suffix. In the composition of the name, social status of the person is also considered. According to Manu Smṛti,[18] the name of a Brāhmana should be auspicious, of a Kṣatriya should denote power, that of a Vaiśya wealth and that of Śūdra contempt.

In Āyurvedic texts, there is provision of two names—Nākṣatrika and Abhiprāyayika.[19] For Nākṣatrika name, it was derived from the name of a Nakṣatra (a lunar auterism). Āśvalāyana Gṛhya Sūtra has similar views.

The naming of a girl has a different basis. The name of a girl should contain an uneven number of syllables. According to Manu,[20] the name of girl should be easy to pronounce, not hard to hear, of clear meaning, charming, auspicious, ending in a long vowel and containing some blessing.

According to Gṛhya Sūtras and Āyurvedic scholars like Caraka,[21] Suśruta[22] and Cakrapāṇi, the Nāmakaraṇa ceremony should be performed on the 10th or the 12th day. But Gobhila Gṛhya Sūtra describe that the naming ceremony should be performed on the 10th, or 100th day or at the end of one year. Vāgbhaṭa[23] is of similar opinion. Bāṇa, in Kādambarī, has also described to perform this ceremony on 10th day.

Caraka has given a detailed description of this ceremony. On 10th day, mother and child should take bath with water purified by drugs, wear clean cloths, ornaments, touch auspicious things, worship god and Brāhmana.

The child is laid down keeping head towards east. Now father of the child prays to god and gives name to the child.[24]

After this ceremony, the infant should be examined very carefully. Normally, the child recovers from various birth traumas including cephalhaematoma, fractures and dislocations, facial palsy and physiological jaundice, etc. Persistence of deformity or jaundice after 10th day should be considered seriously. Thus, this saṃskāra provides opportunity to physician, for proper examination of infant.

3. Niṣkramaṇa (Outing Ceremony)

The custom of this Saṃskāra is very old but in Vedic literature no any reference is available. The Gṛhya Sūtras have described its procedure in very simple way. The child is taken out by his father, with the verse: "That eye," with a look at the sun.[25]

The time for performing the Niṣkramaṇa Saṃskāra, varied from the 12th day to the 4th month of age. The 12th day is recommended by Bhaviṣya Purāṇa. Āyurvedic texts like Kaśyapa Saṃhitā[26] and Aṣṭānga Saṃgraha[27] have advocated it to be performed in the 4th month. The rationale of the option between 3rd and the 4th month is supplied by Yama, who says the ceremony of looking at the sun should be performed in the 3rd, and that of looking at the moon in the 4th month.[28]

Gṛhya Sūtras have advocated that it should be performed by father and the mother, but the paurāṇika and astrological literature extends this privilege to others also. The Viṣṇu Dharmottara, recommends that the solicitions nurse should take the child out.

For performing of the Saṃskāra, a square portion of the court-yard should be smeared with cow-dung and clay, the sign of Svāstika is made on it and grains of rice scattered by the mother. The place should be selected in such way that the sun could be seen. The child after full decoration should be brought to the temple. The child carried out with blowing of Conch-shell and recital of Vedic hymns.

From medical point of view, this ceremony is of great importance.

(i) By exposure to external environment, infant develops resistance power to adjust in different atmosphere.

(ii) By seeing moon/sun, the macular fixation and pupillary adjustment of the child can be observed.

(iii) The reaction of child with the sound produced from bells of temple, may give the clue to rule out hearing defect. After the age of 3 months, the child turns his head towards sound. Control of head may also be observed during visit to temple.

4. Annaprāśana (Feeding of Cereals)

Annaprāśana has very important role in the life of the child. Child receives only milk before this ceremony but due to rapid growth and develop of the chilid, different types of food are required. This ceremony came into practice during the Sūtra period, though references are also available in Veda.

According to Gṛhya Sūtras and Āyurvedic texts,[29] this ceremony should be performed at the age of 5th or 6th month. In Kaśyapa Saṃhitā this Saṃskāra has been described in very detail. According to him, Annaprāśana Saṃskāra should be performed at the age of 10th month and at the age of 6th month there is provision of Phalaprāśan (offering fruit juices) only.[30]

On the day of the feeding ceremony, the material of sacrificial food was cleaned and cooked. After food was prepared, one oblation was offered to speech with the words, "The Gods have generated the goddess, manifold animals speak her forth. May she, the sweet sounding, the highly praised one, come to us, swāhā."[31]

Kaśyapa has described the procedure in detail. On the day of ceremony in Prajāpatya Nakṣatra, cooked food is placed in between the square place prepared by besmearing of cow-dung. The sign of Svāstika is made on it. A pitcher filled with water is also placed there. Physician is the performer of the ceremony. After offering the food to Agni, the remaining part of food is offered to the child, three or five times, Kaśyapa has also mentioned various types of food, beneficial for child.[32]

Most infants gradually reduce the volume and frequency of their demand for breast feeding between 6-12 months of age. As the demand for breast milk decreases, the mother's supply will gradually diminish. Therefore, it is the time when weaning (introduction of supplementary feeding) should be initiated. The prolonged breast feeding after this period may develop rickets, scurvy and anaemia to the child. Thus the Annaprāśana Saṃskāra is not only a religious ceremony but it draws the attention of parents to start supplementary feeding from the stipulated period. The concept of Kaśyapa for Phalaprāśan is more scientific because since both breast as well as cow's milk are poor source of Vit. C. Therefore, it is important that, infant diet must be supplemented with

Vitamin C. Citrus fruits are the best source of Vitamin C. Thus, this ceremony gives a proper time for weaning of the child.

5. Cūḍākaraṇa (Shaving of Head)

The purpose of this saṃskāra is to achieve long and healthy life.[33] Cūḍākaraṇa was a religious ceremony as early as in the Vedic period. Wetting the head for tonsur is mentioned in Atharva Veda.[34] The shaving razor was praised and requested to be harmless.[35]

According to the Gṛhya Sūtras[36] and Manu Smṛti,[37] this ceremony should be performed at the end of the first year or before the expiry of the 3rd year. In the opinion of certain astrological texts, it should be performed only when the Sun is in Uttarāyaṇa.

According to Caraka,[38] cutting and dressing of hair, beard and nails; give strength, vigour, life, purity and beauty. Suśruta opines that shaving and cutting the hair and nails remove impurities and give delight, lightness, prosperity, courage and happiness.[39]

The most important feature of this Saṃskāra is the arrangement of top hairs or śikhā. These top hairs are arranged according to the family custom.[40] Now in the course of evolution, top hair became sign of the Hindus. Hindu sages feel a connection between longevity and the top hair. Ancient Indian surgeon Suśruta has given its explanation. According to him, inside the head near the top, is the joint of a śira and sandhi. Any injury to this part may prove fatal.[41] Top hair are thought to protect this part, thus it provides a prolonged life.

This ceremony provides a chance to examine and care the anterior fontanel. Normally it closes upto the age of 2 years. Delayed closure may be due to cranio-tabes, various serious disorders, like dehydration, meningitis, etc. can be assessed by its examination.

6. Karṇavedhana (Piercing of Ear)

With the beginning of civilization, men used to adorn themselves by wearing of different limbs, especially ears. Atharva Veda[42] has reference for piercing of ear. As a Saṃskāra, Karṇavedhana has its later origin. There is no reference of this ceremony in any Gṛhya Sūtras, except in the Kātyāyana Sūtra incorporated in the appendix of the Pāraskara Gṛhya Sūtra.

Suśruta has mentioned the benefits of this ceremony very clearly. According to him piercing of ears of a child protect him from many diseases.[43] Vāgbhaṭa has also given very detailed description of Karṇavedhana. According to him, this should be performed at the age of 6th, 7th or 8th[44] month but Pāraskara Gṛhya Sūtra advocated it at the age of 3rd or 5th year of life.[45]

For performing the ceremony, an auspicious day especially in winter season should be preferred. The child should be held in the mother's lap. Surgeon should pierce the ears in the middle of the Karṇa-Pīṭha (outer end of the auditory passage) where skin is thinner (Daivakṛta cidra as described by Suśruta) by holding needle in right and ear in the left hand. Right ear should be pierced first in male while in female, left one. Pierced ear should be cared properly otherwise many complications may appear. Vāgbhaṭa has mentioned it in detail.[46]

The trauma produced by piercing the ear, may initiate antigen-antibody reaction, providing active immunity to the child. The place described by Suśruta and Vāgbhaṭa, for piercing the ear is the same, which is used for treating cardio-respiratory problems by Acupuncture.

7. Upanayana Saṃskāra (Threading Ceremony)

This was an important saṃskāra and was performed when a boy was handed over by his father or guardian to the teacher for education. In Atharva Veda[47] the word 'Upanayana' was used for 'accepting the Brahmacārī,' and brahmacārī word was used for a student. In Brāhmaṇa period Upanayana word was used for similar meaning. The motive of this saṃskāra changed time to time but its main intention was education. Later on this saṃskāra become a 'Daihika Saṃskāra' and its main object of education became secondary.

The age of initiation, varied in the case of Brāhmins, Kṣatriyas and Vaiśyas. Gṛhya Sūtra are of opinion that age should be 8 years for Brāhmin, 11 years for Kṣatriyas and 12 years for Vaiśyas.[48] Baudhāyana[49] has given a general range of age and mentioned to perform from the age of 8 to 12 years, depending upon the qualities which he (student) wants to acquire. For performing this Saṃskāra, Manu has advised the age of 5 years for Brāhmaṇas, 6 years for Kṣatriyas and 8 years for Vaiśyas. Difference in age for children of different castes may be due to difference in syllabus of education for children belonging to different groups of caste.

A garment, girdle, and a staff of appropriate materials were then assumed by the student, and he approached to the teacher. The teacher performs the Saṃskāra with 'Sāvitrī Mantra.'

Āyurvedic texts have no reference of this Saṃskāra, however, Suśruta[50] and Vāgbhaṭa[51] have given the time of starting of education, as soon as child becomes fit for this.

According to modern knowledge the brain growth of the child becomes complete, upto the age of 5 years. Therefore, the concept of Manu Smṛti, regarding initiation of this Saṃskāra, is more logical. The thread tied around the waist may serve the purpose to assess the physical growth, to rule out malnutrition.

These above Saṃskāras may be considered as mile-stones of development. By observing these, the physician can assess, the proper growth and development of the child (Table 5).

Table 5: Various childhood saṃskāras and their importance as mile-stones of development

S.N.	*Saṃskāra*	*Period*	*Assessment*
1.	Jātakarma	After birth	Rooting and sucking reflex
2.	Nāmakaraṇa	10th day or 12th or 100th day	Appropriate period for general examination of infants
3.	Niṣkramaṇa	4th month	i. Macular fixation and pupillary adjustment ii. Reaction to sound iii. Head control.
4.	Annaprāśana	6th month or 10th month	i. Appearance of first tooth ii. Functioning of digestive system. iii. Proper time for weaning.
5.	Cūḍākaraṇa	1-3 years	Examination and care of anterior fontanel
6.	Karṇavedhana	6-8 months	A type of active immunization (yukti kṛtabala) initiated with external trauma.
7.	Upanayana	6-8 years	i. Fit for education ii. Assessment of intellect.

REFERENCES

1. Jaiminī Sū. III. 1.3; 2.15; 8.3; IX.2.9
2. Jaiminī Sū. III. 1.3
3. Raghuvaṃśa V. III. 35
4. Kumārasambhava, 10.28
5. Abhijñāna Śākuntalam VII, 23
6. Manu Smṛ. II. 26
7. R.V.III.15.2; II. 26.3
8. A.V.I. 11
9. P.G.S. 10.16; G.G.S. 1.7; A.G.S. 1.15; B.G.S. II.1
10. C.S.Sū. 8.46
11. P.G.S.I. 16.6
12. P.G.S.I. 16, 10-12
13. P.G.S.I. 16.14
14. R.V.X. 55.2; 71.1
15. Ait.Bṛ.I. 3.3
16. Śat.Bṛ.VI. 6.1.3.9
17. P.G.S. I. 17.1
18. Manu Smṛ. II.31
19. C.S.Śā. 8.50
20. Manu Smṛ. II.33
21. C.S.Śā. 8.50
22. S.S.Śā. 10.21
23. A.S.U. 1.27 to 30; A.H.U. 1.22, 23
24. C.S.Śā. 8.50
25. P.G.S.I. 17.5.6
26. K.S.Jāt. 12
27. A.S.U. 1.40
28. Yama. Smṛ.
29. S.S.Śā. 10.49; A.S.Utt. 1.43
30. K.S.Khila. 12

31. P.G.S.I. 19.2
32. K.S.Khil. 12
33. A.G.S.I. 17.12
34. A.V.VI. 68.1
35. Y.V.III. 63
36. P.G.S.II. 1.2
37. Manu.Smṛ. II. 35
38. C.S.Sū .5.99
39. S.S.Ci. 24.72
40. A.G.S.I. 17
41. S.S.Sū.6. 83
42. A.V.VI. 141
43. S.S.Śā. 16.1; S.S.Ci. 19.21
44. A.S.U. 1.144
45. P.G.S. 1.17
46. A.S.U. 1.44-51; A.H.U. 1.28-36
47. A.V. 11.5.3
48. P.G.S. 2.2; A.G.S. 1.19; Sa.G.S. 2.1; B.G.S. 2.5; Āp.G.S. 11; G.G.S. 2.10; Manu. Smr. 2.36; Yaj. Smr. 1.11
49. B.G.S. 2.5.5
50. S.S.Śā. 10.57
51. A.S.U. 1.61

6

Clinical Examination of Children

For the purpose of success in treatment, a physician must know about the general examination of patient. In case of a specialist of children diseases, it has great importance, because children are delicate in nature and unable to explain their comments. It is the child specialist, who makes his diagnosis mainly on the basis of physical examination. Physical examinations are not only necessary for the diagnostic purposes but prediction of longevity of life, future psychological and social status also can be known upto certain extent, by observing it in a way, as described in ancient texts.

Looking at the literature of the ancient period, it is evident that the scholars of that period (particularly Caraka and Kaśyapa), have given much importance to the examinations of children, and their contributions are remarkable.

For the purpose of convenience, the matter of the topic can be subdivided into two headings:

A. General examination of newborns and children

B. Examination of sick children

A. General Examination of Newborn and Children

The main object of physical examination of a healthy newborn, is to decide the life-span. This type of description is available mainly in Caraka Saṃhitā, Suśruta Saṃhitā, Kaśyapa Saṃhitā, Aṣṭānga Saṃgraha and Aṣṭānga Hṛdaya.

Caraka[1] has described that a newborn should be examined after performing nāmakaraṇa saṃskāra, i.e., on 10th day of his birth. This description probably clears the intension of the author that general examination should routinely be performed from 10th day of birth upto its full maturity. By regular examination one may easily detect any physical deformity, various illnesses and proper growth and development. This will help prevention as well as further management of the disease. Caraka has mentioned the following points for examination of children. (Table 6).

The description of Suśruta, regarding physical examination, is mainly related to adults but upto some extent, it can also be applied for children.[2] Because this description is specially not mentioned for children, therefore, has not been included here.

In Kāśyapa Saṃhitā, a separate chapter has been written on certain signs and named 'Lakṣaṇādhyāya.' This chapter deals with auspicious and inauspicious features of the body of children. By the keen observations of these features, one can know about the future life span along with psychological and social status. The child should be examined from downwards to upward, i.e., starting from foot to the end of hair of scalp. The details are as follows:[3]

1. Nails

Different types of nails have their different effect on the life of a child.

(i) Unctuous, thin, smooth and coppery nails indicate that the child will be an administrator in his future life.

(ii) Broad nails—teacher

Table 6: Examination of child (As described by Caraka)

	Body parts		*Findings*	*Remarks*
(A)	**General Observations**	1. Body Hair	Distinct from one another, soft, sparse, oily with firm roots and dark in colour.	Hair growth, nature and colour is influenced by genetic factor.
		2. Skin	Tight and thick	Loose, thin and wrinkled skin is the feature of malnutrition, very prevalent in children.
		3. Voice	Loud, strong and deep	Vocal resonance may be altered during states of diseases like lung consolidation (Bronchopneumonia, etc.), compressed lung tissue (pleural effusion), tuberculous lung cavity.
(B)	**The Head**	1. Cranium or skull	Without defect, well formed slightly larger than usual, yet not disproportionate to the body and resembling an open umbrella is deemed favourable	The skull may be unduly small as in microcephaly or generalised craniostenosis, or unduly large as in hydrocephalus, osteitis deformance, acromegaly or gargoylism, Rachitic head. The average circumference of the skull is 13" at birth, 18" at one year, 20" at 7 and 21" at the age of 15 years.

Body parts		Findings	Remarks
	2. Forehead	Large, compact, levelled well knit with temporal bones, equipped with three vertical lines well developed furnished with horizontal lines, and resembles the half moon	Excessive prominence of the forehead or supraorbital ridges may be due to acromegaly, leontiasis ossium, or to the parrot's node (frontal boosing). Unilateral wrinkling may be due to facial paralysis (Bell's palsy)
(C) **The Eyes**	1. Eyes	Both the eyes should be equal, with well defined parts, with good eye sight and good control over eye ball movement.	In ptosis eyes will appear unequal, also in case of unilateral exophthalmos (in early cases of Grave's disease) cellulitis, orbital haemorrhage, etc. conditions. If there is not proper control over eye balls it may cause deviation of eye. Bitot's spots are found in Vit. A deficiency.
	2. Eye brows	Slightly long, having a small interval in between, equal thick and broad.	Characteristic loss of hair over the outer third or more of the eye brow on either side found in myxo-edema. Patchy hair loss is seen in leprosy.
(D) **The Ear**		Well developed, hairy, broad even, well matched, pendulous, depressed in the back and with large aperture (meatus).	Boils or furuncles, sebaceous cysts, chondromata, local hematomata, cirsoid aneurysms, lupus and other skin disorders are fairly common over the external ear.

Body parts		*Findings*	*Remarks*
(E) **The Nose**		Straight, with nostrils wide enough for large puffs of breath, the tip slightly curved.	Due to congenital deformity, the nose may be unduly long or short, bifurcated, tubular or with a single median eye (cyclopia), saddle nose (depression of nasal bridge) is common in congenital syphilis.
(F) **The Lips**		Lips should be neither thick nor thin endowed with proper breath, cover the mouth properly and red in colour.	Too thick lips are common in acromegaly, myxoedema, cretinism and macrochelia. Thin lips may be racial (as in American Indians) or familial. A common congenital anomaly is harelip (cleft lip). Early cynosis is detectable over the lips.
(G) **The Oral Cavity**	1. Cheek bones	Should be large	
	2. Tongue	Endowed with length and breadth, smooth, thin and without deformity and of pink colour.	A large tongue may be due to congenital macroglossia, acromegaly, myxoedema, cretinism, hurler's; while undue smallness of the tongue may be noted in dehydration, haemorrhage, malnutrition, etc. Change in colour may also indicative of various disorders like anemia, cynosis, fungus infection, etc.

Body parts		Findings	Remarks
	3. Teeth	These should be large and straight.	Normal shape and size may change in various conditions like Hutchinsonian teeth (congenital syphilis), moon malars (deficient development), serrated (malnutrition), pitted (fluorosis).
	4. Palate	Should be smooth, moderately fleshy, warm and red.	Various anomalies of palate like Cleft palate, high arched palate may be observed.
(H) **The Neck**		Neck should not be much long.	Much long is common with a hypo-sthenic constitution, in states of wasting, emaciation, or cachexia, bronchial asthma, pulmonary tuberculosis.
(I) **Flanks**		Should be symmetrical with the shoulders, and must be compact.	Asymmetry may be found in involvement of local muscles, skin lesion and affection of the scapulas.
(J) **Upper Extremities**	1. Shoulder & V. Column	Should be well covered with flesh.	Wasting or loss of flesh is seen in malnutrition. Spinal curvature may present various malpositions like Kyphosis (Parkinsonism, general debility, etc.), scoliosis (may be functional or structural) lordosis (debility, poliomyelitis). Spina bifida is another congenital malformation.

Body parts		*Findings*	*Remarks*
	2. Arms, fingers & hand	Should be rounded, well developed and long. Hand should be large and well developed.	Deformity in shape may be observed in various conditions like Down's syndrome, Hurlers syndrome, Ape hand (muscular atrophy). Fingers should be observed for polydactyly, syndactyly, arachnodactyly, clubbing, etc.
	3. Nails	Nails should be strong, curved, glossy, elevated and convex like a tortoise shell.	The nails become concave hollow and soucer shaped (koylonychia) in iron deficiency anaemia and some times in rheumatic fever and liver diseases.
(K) **Trunk**	1. Chest	Broad and well shaped	Abnormalities in shape may be like—flat chest (rickets), pigeon breast (congenital or rickets), rachitic, barrel chest (Asthma, bronchitis), funnel chest (rickets).
	2. Breast	Should be separate from each other by a wide space.	Less space in between breast may indicate about underlying abnormality of lungs, etc.
	3. Navel	Should be well depressed and with right whorl.	In ascites, umbilicus may become transversely stretched, everted or ballooned out.
	4. Waist	The waist should be thrice the length between the navel and chest, even, not endowed with flesh.	

Body parts		Findings	Remarks
(L) **Lower Extremities**	1. Buttocks	Should be well rounded, compact, fleshy neither very elevated nor very depressed.	In severe malnutrition, there is marked wasting of gluteal fat, causing wrinkling of skin.
	2. Thigh	Thigh should be gradually tapering and well developed.	There are various conditions, in which normal shape of thigh is altered, i.e., coxavara, coxavalga, genuvarum (bow leg), genuvalgum (knock knee),
	3. Calves	These should be neither fleshy nor void of flesh and ending in ankles. Shape should be like that of deer and contain nerves, bones and joints which should be well covered.	In pseudo hypertrophy, the calf muscles appear hypertrophic. Varicose veins, venous thrombosis and deep vein thrombosis are other manifestations.
	4. Feet	Should be convex in shape and like a tortoise shell.	In acromegaly, normal shape is changed. Talipus equinovarous and flat foot are other complications.
	5. Heel	Heel should be neither very fleshy nor void of flesh.	

(iii) Nails having vertical ridges—long life

(iv) Dry nails—sorrow

(v) Flower like white spots on nails—thief or robber

(vi) Circular white spots on nails—short life span.

White nails with normal texture (leuconychia) are of four major types—total, partial, striate and punctate. All but the punctate or may be hereditary and all four forms may be acquired. The total and partial forms usually follow a severe long lasting systemic disorder or local insult. This is most commonly seen in hepatic cirrhosis but is also reported in typhoid fever, exposure to extreme cold, ulcerative colitis and trauma from nail biting. Leuconychia striata may follow a short or recurrent systemic disorder or local trauma. This is seen in severe chronic hypoalbuminaemia due to chronic renal disease, MI, cardiac insufficiency, pneumonia, Hodgkin's diseases. Leuconychia punctata, white patches on the nails is very common and has no clinical significance. It is often results from minor trauma to the nail matrix.

(vii) Cracked nails—not independent.

(viii) Discoloured nails—addicted to vices.

(ix) Nails bented forward with shape of pearl-oyster—poverty.

Blue nails may result from administration of mepacrine. Red half-moons may be seen in congestive cardiac failure. Multiple pigmented spots may occur in addisons disease.

(x) Small rounded and prominent nails which are well fixed into skin—happy life.

(xi) Large nails—middle life.

(xii) Broad, white and irregular nails - wanderer.

Broad or square nails occur in acromegaly and cretinism. Long and narrow nails may be observed in hypopituitarism and cunuchodism. Parrot beak nails are seen with finger clubbing.

2. Feet

(i) A well developed foot with vertical lines—long life, wealthy and will be chief or leader.

(ii) Sole of the foot having any one of the following signs will be a king—Svastika, plough, lotus, Śaṅkha (Conch-Shell), wheel, horse, elephant and chariot.

(iii) Coppery and smooth feet—lucky.

(iv) Twisted feet—medium life.

Talipas equinovarus (club foot) is a common deformity of the foot of congenital origin but sometimes secondary to neurological diseases, with both feet adducted downwards and inwards with a medial concavity. The other varieties of talipas (viz. equinus, varus, valgus and calcaneus) are much less common.

(v) White feet—poor

(vi) Sole devoid of lines—servant

(vii) Sole having too much lines—patient.

In acromegaly, the skin and subcutaneous tissue are thickened, therefore, sole gives appearance of too much lines than a normal feet.

(viii) Round and smooth heels—possessing all good qualities.

(ix) Small heels—short life span and without children.

(x) Flat foot—one who is after other's wives.

Pes planus (flat foot) is a common and bilateral frequent congenital deformity of the foot, caused by a loss of the longitudinal arch of the foot and resulting in adduction and eversion of the foot at the midtarsal joint.

It is very difficult to explain the effect of flat foot mentioning by Kaśyapa, but anyhow it indicate that the Kaśyapa has very keen observation and drawn the attention of another physicians to examine the feet.

(xi) Long finger, nails and feet—long life.

(xii) Short fingers, nails and feet—short life.

3. Fingers

(i) Child having strong fingers—long life.

(ii) Obscure (gūḍa) interphallangeal joints—pleasure seeking.

(iii) Corpulent (sthūla) interphallangeal joints—teacher.

(iv) Fingers with hair—poor life.

Acute gout classically starts in the great toe, which become swollen, red, shiny and painful.

4. Heel

(i) Rough, thin, irregular, cracked and dirty heel—bad life.

Foots of the child, if are not kept clean then due to ringworm infection, it may become rough with cracking, which is extremely painful.

5. Dorsum of Foot

(i) Well developed dorsum of foot without prominent veins or hair—good life.

(ii) Underdeveloped dorsum of foot with much hair and prominent veins—thief.

Too much prominent veins may develop as vericose ulcers in future.

6. Gulpha (Ankles)

(i) A child having strong, small, hairless and less prominent veins—good

(ii) Too much prominent ankle—loss of wealth

(iii) Too big or broad ankle—sorrowful life.

Ankles are the best region, where early oedema may be detected.

7. Prajanghā (Lower Part of Leg)

(i) Thin lower part of legs are considered good for life.

(ii) Large lower part of legs are considered bad for spouse, children, wealth, happiness and the child may be thief in future.

Bowing of lower leg (rickets), knock-knee (congenital, ricket or ill-health) are common deformities of lower leg. Large lower leg may be feature of philariasis.

8. Janghā (Legs)

(i) Well-developed legs without hair and prominent veins—good.

(ii) Wasted or bulky and with much hairs and prominent veins—bad life and may lose their spouse.

In children wasting of legs, is the feature of malnutrition.

9. Jānu (Knees)

Strong knee joints are considered good. Rheumatic fever and septic arthritis are the condition in which knee joints are affected very commonly.

10. Uru (Thighs)

Muscular, smooth thighs without visible veins are good.

Atrophy of muscle of thigh may be due to nutritional deficiency or due to neurological or muscular involvement. Lymphadenopathy of this region (inguinal) my be due to septic infection etc. conditions.

11. Sphika (Buttocks)

(i) Rounded but not oblong, without any scar and hairs and symmetrical buttocks are good.

(ii) Wasted or thin buttocks—childless in future.

(iii) Long buttocks—loses his importance.

(iv) Big buttocks—sexy.

(v) Small buttocks—with good character.

The nutritional status of muscle, whether soft, flabby and wasted should be carefully assessed by inspection and palpation. The size of muscles varies with age, sex, body build, state of nutrition.

12. Kukundara (Ischial Tuberosity)

(i) Deep, hairless, divided and symmetrical are good.

(ii) Kukundara with hairs—wanderer.

(iii) With spirals toward right side—good.

(iv) Big in size indicating—long life.

(v) Narrow indicate the short life span.

13. Jaghana (Pelvis)

Circumference of pelvis and chest should be equal, but in boys, the chest circumference should be greater than of buttock, while buttocks circumference should be greater than chest in girls. Opposite measurement is not considered good.

Kaśyapa has mentioned anthropometric measurement of chest and pelvis. Any change in it may indicate towards improper growth and development.

14. Vṛṣaṇa (Testicles)

Kaśyapa has correlated the complexion of the boy with characteristics of testicles. In children with white complexion, scrotum is big and hanging, while the colour of scrotum is dark in dark children and whitish in children of pink complexion. Other features and their effects are as follows:

(i) Pink and hairy scrotum — Medium life

(ii) Well-developed — Good life

(iii) Thin or underdeveloped — Bad life, impotence or sterility, short life span and sorrowful life.

Small and shrunken testicles and epididymis, with atrophy, may either result from infectious, fevers, such as mumps; injuries; torsion of the spermatic cord; or represent a congenital malformation. Undescended testicle (Cryptochism) is an another congenital deformity with defective descent of one or both testicles. These conditions may ultimately leads to impotence or sterility.

Shape of scrotum or testes resembling that of bullock, ass, goat and sheep are lucky, good and indicative of long life.

15. Prajanana (Śepha)—(Penis)

Soft, long, erectile, well developed penis with pink glans and sufficient urethral opening is considered good while short and thin, and too much long, hairless, having spiral on left side and with whitish or blackish discharges is considered bad and incapable of producing child.

Purulent urethral discharge is highly suggestive of gonorrhoeal urethritis.

16. Urine

If the child void without trouble, stream is not too thin, urine is not less in quantity and flow is good then these features indicate that child is normal. Urine having bad odour, passing with pain (dysuria), too hot and discolouration are not good features. Besides this if urine is passed at indefinite times and without producing sound at the time of voiding, is also bad. After voiding, if the urine spread on the ground in various directions then it indicate that boy/girl will be childless in future.

The above features, mentioned by Kaśyapa are actually urinary tract symptoms which includes dysuria, frequency of urination, retention of urine, hematuria etc. These are common in renal calculus and urinary tract infection.

17. Yoni (Vagina)

Description of yoni is given in much detail. Different features and their effects are as follows:

(i) Vagina having cart like shape—good for child birth.
(ii) Broad shaped—good luck
(iii) Long in shape—abortion and miscarriage
(iv) Rounded—prostitute
(v) Bulging out—no children
(vi) Narrow vaginal opening (Sūcīmukhī)—bad luck.
(vii) Too much wide, dry, long, irregular and without clitoris (linga)—physical and mental sorrow.
(viii) Well placed—bears more girls.
(ix) Bulging, fleshy and well shaped—bears boys.
(x) Excessive hairy—widow.
(xi) Neither very prominent nor very deep and with rows of hair on both sides—good.
(xii) Bulky with dense and excessive hair—Indulges in sex with many men.
(xiii) Depressed vagina—bad luck.
(xiv) Anteriorly placed—average.

18. Kukṣhi (Flanks)

(i) Prominent kukṣhi—normal.
(ii) Hairy—wanderer
(iii) With prominent veins—desire for bad food
(iv) Under developed or concave—desire for bad food.
(v) Even—average
(vi) Right flank more prominent than left—bears son.

(vii) Left flank more prominent than right—bears daughter.

19. Udara (Abdomen)

(i) Slightly prominent, not lax, not bulky or hard abdomen—long life.

(ii) Dry and sunken abdomen—poverty.

(iii) Prominent abdomen—enjoy life.

(iv) Large and irregular abdomen—mixed character and enjoyment.

(v) Wasted abdomen—no children.

(vi) Lower abdomen without prominent veins or skin folds—short life span.

(vii) Abdomen depressed above umbilicus—short life span.

Kaśyapa has mentioned the effect of various types of abdominal contour. There are three main types of abdominal contour. The flat type of abdomen is common in young adults. Globular or round type presents usually through obesity or lack of muscle tone. Scaphoid or boat shaped abdomen is common in thin subjects and those suffering from wasting diseases, cachexia, dehydration and meningitis.

Prominence of the superficial veins of the abdominal wall is abnormal, and indicative of obstruction to the return circulation through the portal vein or the inferior vena cava. This may result from an enlarged liver, intra-abdominal tumour, chronic distension of the stomach or mediastinal new growth.

On examination of abdomen one or more lines or skin folds can be observed. Number of these lines have their own importance.

Number of lines/skin-folds	*Significance*
(i) One	Good
(ii) Two	Intelligent
(iii) Three	Lucky
(iv) Four	Long life and more children
(v) Many	Bad life.

Few lines over abdomen are normal while too much lines (white), the so called linear albicans are evidence of stretching of skin through ascites, abdominal tumor, cyst, massive enlargement of spleen, rapid weight gain and in Cushing's syndrome. Purplish straie over the abdomen are suggestive of adrenocortical hyperfunction of Cushing's syndrome.

20. Nābhi (Umbilicus)

(i) Deep, turned towards right, rounded, slightly elevated, prominent edges, and without hair or prominent veins—normal and good.

(ii) Spiral like and unprominent edges—missed life (happiness and sorrow).

(iii) Small umbilicus—no child.

(iv) Abnormally situated (displaced from its site)—wanderer.

(v) Large, deep and with prominent edges—ruler or administrator.

Normally indrawn or flush with the skin surface, the umbilicus may alter in shape or position, depending on the tone of the abdominal muscles and the degree of abdominal distension. In ascites, it may become transversely stretched, averted or baloon out.

21. Gudā (Anus)

Features of gudā are similar to that of nābhi.

The anus should be examined for normalcy of position and for intrinsic disorders such as stenosis, paralysis or fissure. Prolapse, if present, will be obvious.

22. Pārśva

(i) Rounded, fleshy, smooth, hairless and without prominent veins—normal and good.

(ii) With hairs and prominent veins—wanderer.

23. Praṣṭhadeśa (Back)

(i) Even, broad in upper part without prominent veins and hairs or whorls of hair—good

(ii) Depression in middle—long life.

(iii) Curved (spinal deformity)—sorrow.

(iv) Small area—short life.

(v) Hairy—without friends and very few children.

Kaśyapa has mentioned very rightly about the normal spinal curvature. The normal spine displays a mild convexity of the thoracic spine, a mild concavity of the cervical spine and a definite concavity of the lumbar spine, without any lateral curvature. Abnormal spinal curvature may be due to various disorders like kyphosis (due to rheumatoid arthritis, general debility, Parkinsonism or growth disturbance of bones); Scoliosis (due to poliomyelitis, rickets, congenital); lordosis (due to general debility, wasting disease, poliomyelitis, faulty posture).

24. Skandha (Shoulders)

(i) Hairy shoulders—seller, labour carrying weight on shoulder and painter.

(ii) Wasted shoulders—poor, wanderers.

(iii) Unctuous—farmer.

(iv) Well developed—rich.

(v) Firm shoulders—brave.

(vi) Loose—weak.

(vii) Prominent shoulder—good.

(viii) Prominent shoulders in girls, depressed shoulders in boys—bad.

In dislocation of shoulder, it shows an abnormality of position with flaccid hanging of the arm, limitation of movement and wasting of muscle near shoulder. This condition may be congenital or acquired (injury or acute poliomyelitis).

25. Kakṣhā (Axilla)

(i) Prominent, broad, well developed and well differentiated kakṣhā is good. Having opposite qualities is bad.

(ii) Excessive hairs in girls—bad.

Axilla must always be examined for lymphadenopathy. These may be due to septic infections of the upper extremity, shoulder, back or breast, tuberculosis or lymphatic leukaemia.

26. Bāhu (Arms)

(i) Well shaped with strong elbows and touching the knees are good.

(ii) Arms having visible prominent veins—long life.

(iii) Hairy arms—many children.

(iv) Arms having no any visible vein—childless.

(v) Arms having zig-zag veins—hard life.

(vi) Mole on arms—wanderer.

(vii) Big moles on arm—quarrelsome.

27. Maṇibandha (Wrist)

Wrist of boys should be strong while thin in case of girls.

When hand is slightly flexed, few lines appears on wrist. These lines have their importance, according to number.

No. of lines		*Significance in the life of child*
(i)	2 or 3 broken lines	Good
(ii)	First line unbroken	Wealth
(iii)	Second and third line unbroken	Important person
(iv)	Third line unbroken	Long life and many children.
(v)	Four lines unbroken	Rājarṣi (Royal)
(vi)	Five or six lines unbroken	100 children
(vii)	Seven line unbroken	Divine person
(viii)	Even if one line is unbroken	Happy life
(ix)	All the lines without break, unctuous, clear and deep	Administrator

Modern texts have not mentioned any condition in which such lines are considered for diagnosis.

28. Hair

Before the description of hair, some portion of original text is missing. Probably this may contain the description of lines appearing on palm (palmistry).

(i) In women, too much long and too much short hairs are considered bad.

(ii) Scalp should be smooth, clean and scarless.

In the case of child suffering from Kwashiorkar have changes in their hair. The hair is sparse, thin and losses its elasticity. The colour of the hair becomes brownish with golden-yellow ends.

29. Gait

(i) Gait like elephant, ox, lion and tiger—king.
(ii) Slow moving—good.
(iii) Fast moving—suffering with pleasure and sorrow quickly.
(iv) Person having oblique gait—not good.
(v) Stammering gait—bad.

A normal gait may become abnormal as the result of muscle power, alteration of muscle tone, inco-ordination of movement, deformity, pain during movement or hysteria. The majority of abnormal gait are due to diseases of the nervous system or of the muscle.

30. General Features

Along with above mentioned examination, specific parts of the body should also be noted for some general features:

(i) Cut body parts—bad
(ii) Too white or dark complexion—bad.
(iii) Too tall or too short stature—bad.
(iv) Too thin or too obese body—bad.
(v) Excessive or hairless body—bad.
(vi) Too flabby or too hard body—bad.

Caraka has also mentioned these features under "Aṣṭanindatīya" Chapter (Eight Bad Features). Normal body structure will lead to a good health. Excess or deficiency of any body part or organ may be pathological condition and disturb the normal health and life of a person.

Caraka has given the qualities of normal body parts, while Kaśyapa has mentioned normal as well as abnormal features and their probable effect on future life of the child. These features may reveal various status of life and may be explained from modern knowledge, however, other features giving clues about the future social, psychological and physical status of the child. It is based on observations of ancient scholars. Therefore, it is an unique contribution of their in this field because others have not given such descriptions for future prediction of physical, psychological as well as social status of a man.

Besides these, some indirect references are also available. The scholars have described several procedures like purification of mouth, massage, bath, care of bregma, etc. which is to be performed in newborns.[4] During these procedures, one may detect congenital malformations during purification of mouth (mukha sodhana), abnormalities of lips and oral cavity, hare lip, tongue tie, cleft and high arched palate and presence of congenital tooth, etc. may be observed. Care of bregma (by taila picu) may provide opportunity to examine skull for anterior fontanel and birth injuries like caput succidanum.

B. Examination of Children for Diagnosis (To know the Ailments of Children)

Weeping is a normal phenomenon of children, especially of infants. Cry of a ill child differs from a normal one. An expert may very well understand the problem of the child by this clue. Beside this, the activities of the ill child indicate towards the problem of the child. It requires good skill and knowledge of the subject. Ancient texts like Suśruta Saṃhitā,[5] Kaśyapa Saṃhitā,[6] Aṣṭānga Saṃgraha,[7] Aṣṭānga Hṛdaya,[8] Mādhava Nidāna,[9] Gada Nigraha[10] and Vangasena Saṃhitā[11] have ample references which give detailed informations regarding the diagnostic methods. Suśruta[12] has mentioned that the ill child repeatedly touches the affected body parts and cries. If child is suffering from the disease of Mūrdhā (head), he is unable to open his eyes and looses head control. Pain in Vasti (urinary bladder) causes retention of urine, dysurea, thirst and coma; gastro-intestinal tract disorders cause retention of urine and stool, discolouration, vomiting, distension of abdomen and rumbling sound in abdomen.

Kaśyapa Saṃhitā contains a separate chapter, describing signs and symptoms of various disorders and named 'Vedanādhyāya.' In this chapter Vṛddha Jīvaka has asked Kaśyapa about the methods of diagnosis of diseases of ill children, as most of them are unable to explain their complaints. Kaśyapa has explained the answer very comprehensively. Manifestations of signs (diseases) of various sites, as described by Kaśyapa[13] are mentioned hereunder in a systematic manner.

General Signs/Symptoms

1. *Śirah śūla (Headache)*

In headache the child may have following manifestations:

(i) Excessive movement of head.

(ii) Closes his eyes.

(iii) Sudden weeping in night, while sleeping in day.

(iv) Anoxia and insomnia.

Headache is a common symptom in childhood. The commonest cause of headache before puberty is migraine or an acute infection. Other common causes of headache are— a stuffy room, lack of fresh air, climatic condition, hunger and emotional factors.

2. *Jvara (Fever)*

Child may have following prodromal signs:

(i) Repeated contraction of extremities, yawning and coughing.

(ii) The child suddenly embraces the mother/wet-nurse and dislikes to suck breast.

(iii) Excessive salivation.

(iv) Body becomes warm and discoloured. Forehead is also warm.

(v) Child develops anorexia and his feet become cold.

The following conditions are present in fever:

Normal variation, dehydration, overheating, malingering, child abuse, infections, etc. McCarthy and Dolan (1976), in a study found the causes in order were—pneumonia, otitis media, meningitis, septicemia, pharyngitis, dehydration, cellulitis, and unknown causes.

3. *Triṣṇā (Thirst)*

(i) Child is not satisfied even after excessive breast feeding thus he cries.

(ii) Dryness of lips and fontanelle (Tālu) is depressed.

(iii) Anxious for taking water.

The above features are of mild dehydration.

4. *Kāmalā (Jaundice)*

The colour of eyes (conjuctiva) nails, mouth (mucous membrane), stool and urine become yellowish.

In Pāṇḍu and Kāmalā, child loses his enthusiasm, having loss of appetite and body requires blood.

In infancy jaundice may be due to deficiency of the enzyme glucoronyl transferase (physiological, breast milk induced, Cigler-Najjar-Syndrome, Gilberts disease), increased bilirubin production (congenital haemolytie disease e.g. ABO & Rh incompatibility, drugs like Vit. K, etc. infections, absorption of blood from a large cephalhaematoma or other haemorrhage) and obstructive jaundice (neonatal hepatitis, biliary atresia, cystic fibrosis). Jaundice after infancy may be due to obstruction (infective hepatitis), cirrhosis of liver, Wells disease and infectious mononucleosis.

5. *Pāṇḍu (Anaemia, pallor)*
   - (i) Oedema around umbilical region.
   - (ii) Eyes, nails and mouth become whitish.
   - (iii) Decreased digestive power.
   - (iv) Oedema of periorbital region.

Many children are treated for anaemia in general practice when there is no anaemia at all. The child may be pale because he has been indoors a good deal, is tired, or has an infection, or because he has a pale complexion. Mild degree of anaemia can not be detected without proper laboratory investigations. The causes of anaemia may be blood loss, nutritional defects, infection, haemolysis, defective red cell production and other serious blood diseases. Oedema may be due to associated protein deficiency.

Symptoms Related to Ear and Eye Disorders

1. *Karṇa Vedanā (Pain in ears)*
   - (i) Child touches ears.
   - (ii) Excessive movements of head.
   - (iii) Nausea and anorexia.

2. *Insomnia*

The usual cause of ear pain is acute otitis media, especially, if, temperature is raised. Other causes are as follows:

- (i) The pinna—injury, boil, herpes.
- (ii) Ext. auditory meatus—boil, foreign body, herpes, otitis, external injury.
- (iii) Referred pain from lower molar teeth, temporo-mandibular joint, throat, possibly cervical spine, mumps.

The features mentioned by Kaśyapa are: excessive movement of head, nausea, anorexia and secondary due to pain.

3. *Cakṣu-roga (Disorders of Eye)*

The child suffering from any disorder of eye may have following features:

(i) Difficulty in vision.
(ii) Pain, itching, inflammation and redness of eyes.
(iii) Excessive lachrymation.
(iv) Sticky eyes (especially on sleeping).

Symptoms related to the Mouth and Throat

1. *General symptoms of mouth (Mukha roga)*

(i) Excessive salivation.
(ii) Excessive movements of head.
(iii) Nausea and anorexia.
(iv) Insomnia.

These are general symptoms of any problem related to mouth and throat.

2. *Kaṇṭha Vedanā (Pain in Throat)*

(i) Vomiting/regurgitation of milk.
(ii) Constipation due to use of articles increasing śleṣmā.
(iii) Mild fever, aversion from food and nausea.

Infectious mononucleosis may cause pharyngitis or tonsillitis with exudate or membrane. Diptheria may be strongly suspected because of the membrane, but the diagnosis had to be confirmed in the laboratory.

3. *Adhijihvikā roga (Diseases of epiglottis)*

(i) Excessive salivation, aversion from food and nausea.
(ii) Inflammation and pain on cheecks and child used to keep open his mouth.

These features are due to acute epiglottitis, occurs predominantly in the 2 to 7 year-old group. The child may have high fever, dyspnoea, dysphagia, salivation and low pitched stridor due to obstruction.

4. *Kaṇṭhaśotha (Pharyngitis)*
   (i) Inflammation of throat.
   (ii) Fever, disliking of food.
   (iii) Headache.

Symptoms Related to Gastro-intestinal Tract

1. *Atisāra (Diarrhoea)*

The child may have following prodromal features:
   (i) Discolouration of body.
   (ii) Feeling of dullness, nausea and insomnia.
   (iii) Defective function of Vāta.

Discolouration of body and feeling of dullness may be due to dehydration. Due to defective function of vāta there is hypermotality of GIT, causing diarrhoea. This may be psychogenic or due to food poisoning or due to toxins of various bacteria.

2. *Visūcikā (Gastroenteritis)*
   (i) Burning sensation and pain like piercing by needles.
   (ii) Difficulty in breathing and pain in cardiac region.

Visūcikā is an acute disease of the gastro-intestinal tract and has symptoms like gastroenteritis. In the above description, Kaśyapa has not mentioned about nature of stool, however, the sign and symptoms denote electrolyte imbalance due to excessive diarrhoea and vomiting. The features resemble with hyponatremia and acidosis.

3. *Alasaka (Paralytic ileus)*

(i) Loss of head control and feeling of piercing sensation.

(ii) Repeated yawning, disliking of breast feeding, vomiting and distention of abdomen (ādhmāna).

Kaśyapa opines that differentiation of Visūcikā and Alasaka is some times very difficult.

Diarrhoeal disorders may lead to dehydration along with electrolyte imbalance and especially loss of potassium (Hypokalemia) presents the features of Alasaka.

5. *Ānāha*

(i) Eyes are widely opened.

(ii) Pain in joints and feeling of dullness.

(iii) Retention of urine, vāyu and stool.

Ānāha may develop, if Alasaka is persistent. It is a symptom rather than a disease. Obstruction of stool is due to constipation, which may be associated with any disease (imperforated anus, anorectal stenosis, Hirschsprung's disease, secondary to paralytic ileus, etc.) or without any disease (bottle fed disease, unwise toilet training). Faecal impaction is one of the major cause resulting in retention of urine. Other symptoms like wide opened eye, pain in joints, feeling of dullness and fatigue may be associated with the above problems.

6. *Cardiroga (Vomiting)*

The child have following prodromal features:

(i) Belching without any apparent cause.

(ii) Feeling of excessive sleep and yawning.

A common cause of significant regurgitation in a young infant is faulty feeding technique. In the newborn infant, vomiting should suggest congenital obstruction of the digestive tract, particularly if the emesis is bile stained. After several weeks hypertrophic pyloric stenosis should be considered. Vomiting, particularly in babies, can occur with any illness, but central nervous system lesions, and infections, especially gastroenteritis are common causes. Later in childhood, the acute abdomen is a common cause of vomiting.

7. *Udara Śūla (Pain in abdomen or intestinal colic)*
   (i) Refuses breast feeding and cry.
   (ii) Sleeps on back and abdomen becomes stupefied.
   (iii) Rigor and swelling on face.

This is one of the most common complaint of childhood. A young infant who cries is considered hungry, but if, crying persists after feeding, the infant is thought to be in agony. Infantile colic is a common phenomenon that causes young infants to cry for prolonged periods, usually at any time of day or night. The serious disorders that cause abdominal pain and require urgent attention in young infants are acute enteritis and strangulated bowel. In pre-schoolers and older children, appendicitis and urinary tract infections are common causes of pain.

Symptoms Related to Anorectal Disorders

Arśa (*Haemorroids*)

(i) Child becomes weak and passes solid stool mixed with blood.
(ii) Pain and itching in anus.

Hemorrhoids are uncommon in infants and children, however, anal fissure is a common acquired lesion in infancy. Pain on defecation is a main manifestation. Bright red blood on the surface of the stool and a history of prolapse of something suggests rectal polyp.

Symptoms Related to Respiratory Tract

1. *Pīnasa* (*Coryza*)

The child may have following complaints:

(i) Breathing from mouth at the time of breast feeding.

(ii) Nasal discharges, warm forehead, and repeated coughing and sneezing.

Even the youngest babies may develop cold, and the common complication of it is otitis media. Other complications include laryngitis and bronchopneumonia. The baby may have difficulty in breathing and may have some difficulty in feeding because of blockade of the nose. The child may be febrile with complaints of coughing, if complication occurs.

2. *Śvāsa roga*

The following prodromal features may appear:

(i) Exhalation of excessive warm air during respiration.

(ii) Sudden welching in weak child may precipitate hiccough.

Hiccough occurs in young babies, frequently after feed. The other causes of hiccough include subphrenic abscess, diaphragmatic pleurisy, cerebral tumour, peritonitis or uraemia. It may follow respiratory tract infection and difficulty in breathing.

Symptoms Related to Nervous System/Psychological Disorders

1. *Unamāda (Insanity)*

Child develops delirium and upset of mind.

2. *Apasmāra (Hysteria)*

Child suddenly makes abnormal sound like a horse.

3. *Madātyaya (Effect of Sedatives or Alcoholic Products)*
   (i) The child loses his consciousness and suffer from insomnia.
   (ii) Complaints of vomiting, disliking wet-nurse, feeling of uneasiness, confusion, fear, anxiety and thirst confirms the diagnosis of madātya.

The all above conditions, mentioned by Kaśyapa seems to be disorders of emotion, especially neurosis. According to psychoanalytic theory, psychoneurosis arises from intrapsychlic conflict between one's wishes for expression of sexual and aggressive drives and the prohibitions of the conscience against these expressions. Anxiety can be expressed as irratibility or whimpering, or as worry in older children. It can also appear as a phobia, such as fear of the dark or of going outside. Sometimes anxiety is converted into a somatic symptoms or a conversion reaction such as paralysis of a limb or the reproduction of a convulsive disorder.

The over anxious child is upset beyond apparent reason. There may be excessive shyness, shaking, frequent crying, insomnia, tics and so on. Children with hysterical neurosis are able to achieve massive repression of certain ego states without overt evidence of anxiety.

Symptoms Related to Uro-Genital Disorders

1. *Mūtrakriccha (Dysuria)*
   (i) Feeling of a type of excitement (romaharṣa and angaharṣa) and pain during micturation.
   (ii) Biting of lips.
   (iii) Touches supra-pubic area (Basti pradeśa).

During and after micturation pain is felt in the urethra and sometimes in supra pubic region. Its presence suggests irritation of mucosa of the bladder or urethra like acute urethritis, acute cystitis, bladder-stone, etc.

2. *Aśmarī (Bladder Stone)*

   (i) If crystals/gravels are present in urine, the child have increased frequency of micturation.

   (ii) Pain during micturation. Child excessively cries and become very weak.

Pain during micturation is a prominent feature of stone in bladder. Sometimes dribbling of urine may be associated with it. Glycosurea may be due to excessive blood glucose levels as in diabetes mellitus or to defective renal tubular reabsorption—renal glycosurea a specific hereditary defect. Kaśyapa has mentioned about glycosurea as a symptom of aśmarī, however, there is no correlation between urinary calculi and glycosurea.

Symptoms Related to Skin Disorders

1. *Śuṣka Kaṇḍū (Pruritis)*

   (i) Itching sensation, specially in night.

   (ii) Child cries and scratches the body parts.

2. *Ārdra Kaṇḍū*

Śuṣka Kaṇḍū in due course convert into ārdra kaṇḍū. Child feels pleasure on scratching but on excessive scratching, discharges appear which are associated with pain and burning sensation.

Pruritis or itching can be defined simply as a desire to scratch. It is the singlemost important dermatological symptom. Generalised pruritis may be due to allergy, skin diseases (scabies, lichen planus, dermatitis herpetiformis), systemic disease (diabetes mellitus, obstructive jaundice, etc.), psychogenic and use of certain drugs (due to drug allergy).

3. *Visarpa (Erysipelas)*

   (i) Reddish circular spots appear on the body of the child.

   (ii) Child suffers from thirst, burning, fever and uneasiness and like to take sweet and cold articles.

The above features of visarpa are similar to the erysipelas, celulitis with acute lymphangitis of the skin which spread marginally. The skin is erythematous and indurated, the margins of the lesions have arised firm border. The skin lesion is usually asociated with fever, vomiting and irritability. These symptoms subside when progression of the rash ceases. It is a highly fatal condition and may produce various complications.

4. *Jantu-Daṃśa (Insect bite)*

Healthy baby loses his sleep at night and red spots appear on any part of the body, confirm the diagnosis of insect bite.

In night, mostly mosquitoes, lice and bucks, etc. may bite the child. These insects introduce saliva into the skin while sucking. This foreign protein produces allergic manifestation including rashes or blister formation.

Symptoms Related to Graha (Infectious Diseases)

(a) *General Features*

Kaśyapa has mentioned following common features of Graha roga:

   (i) The child suffers from fever, there is aversion from food and salivation.

   (ii) Difficulty in breathing.

(b) *Fatal Signs*

The following features in wet-nurse indicate the possibility of death of child (nursed by her):

(i) The wet-nurse sees bad dreams.

(ii) Milk comes out of her breast automatically and she forgets her baby.

(iii) The child suddenly falls from the lap of mother/wet-nurse.

(c) *Prodermal Features of Graha Roga*

(i) Hagged birds make their nest near the sleeping child.

(ii) Cat jumps over child and like the offspring.

(iii) Bad smell from body and mouth, excrementation on the tip of nose and mother and child bear red coloured and inauspicious garlands in dreams.

(iv) Child suffer from fear and his behaviour changes.

He also receives less food and normalcy of the excretion of urine and stool is disturbed.

(v) Loss of head control and involuntary movements of extremities.

(vi) Child complaints of thirst and feels sleepy.

The child having above complaints may be suffering from graha roga.

Other Symptoms

1. *Uroghāta (Injury of chest wall)*

Child may have complaints similar to Pīnasa roga (breathing from mouth while feeding, nasal discharges, warm forehead, repeated coughing and sneezing) along with exhalation of warm air.

Injury to the chest wall may cause fracture of ribs, which leads to various other complications like pneumothorax, haemothorax, etc. In the neonate, over enthusiastic resuscitation or difficult labour may be complicated with injury of chest wall, producing pneumothorax.

Symptoms Related to Metabolic Disorders

1. *Āmadoṣa*

   (i) Child becomes clammy and feels aruchi, nidrā, pāṇḍu and arati.

   (ii) Aversion from playing, food, sleep and child also dislikes the wet-nurse.

   (iii) If child has taken bath, he still appears dirty and vice versa.

Āmadoṣa is a complex condition and may be simulated with various conditions characterised by sweating, pallor, fatigue, nervousness (occur as a result of excessive secretion of epinaphrine in response to hypoglycemia), irritability, negativism, alterations in behaviour and psychotic behaviour, etc. (due to CNS dysfunction).

2. *Prameha*

   (i) Feeling of heavyness and dullness of body.

   (ii) Sudden passing of urine.

   (iii) Flies like to sit over the area of ground where urine has been passed.

   (iv) Urine becomes whitish and ghana (specific gravity is increased).

Prameha is a symptom of various renal diseases (21 including diabetes). The prameha mentioned in Vedanādhyāya of Kaśyapa Saṃhitā has features of Diabetes mellitus of Juvenile origin. The most frequent symptoms are polyurea, nocturea. In addition, weightloss, symptoms of fatigue, irritability and moodiness may be part of the initial symptom complex.

Kaśyapa has mentioned few points for urine test of diabetic child. Attraction of flies for urine is due to much presence of sugar in urine. Colour and specific gravity is also changed of such urine.

These all above mentioned features are mainly prodromal signs/symptoms of various diseases. Early diagnosis of a disease is always helpful to physician to cure the ill child very well in their early stage because these diseases, in their later course may prove fatal or difficult to treat. Due to this fact, Kaśyapa has given the description of signs and symptoms of various disorders very vividly.

Vāgbhaṭa has given very short description about diagnostic aspect of children and prodromal features of very few disorders like abdominal discomforts, diseases of uro-genital tract and headache have been mentioned. If the child excessively cries and/or having bad facial expressions it may be considered that the child is suffering from any general disorder of the body.[14]

Treatise of later period, like Mādhava Nidāna, Vangasena and Gada Nigraha also contain some descriptions for diagnosis of children disorders, but these have followed only their previous texts. No special contribution has been made by these texts, in this field, except Kaśyapa.

REFERENCES

1. C.S.Śā. 8.51
2. S.S.Sū .35.1-17
3. K.S.Sū .28.1-6
4. C.S.Śā. 8.42-46; S.S.Śā. 10.11,12; A.S.Śā. 3.37
5. S.S.Śā. 10.39-41
6. K.S.Sū.Vedanā. 25.1-52
7. A.S.U. 2.9
8. A.H.U. 2.5-8
9. M.N. 68.4-7
10. V.S. 70.7
11. G.N. 11.5-8
12. S.S.Śā. 10.39-41
13. K.S.Sū.Vedanā. 25
14. A.S.U. 2.9

7

Principles of Treatment and Drug Therapy in Children

The treatment of children is very arduous job for physician because children are of delicate nature and are incapable to express their problems. Their doṣas are also not stable. Due to these reasons the physician has to handle them with his specialized knowledge and experience. One should be also careful regarding the prescription of drugs to children. The drug should be prescribed by keeping in mind about the nature of disease and child itself.[1]

General Principles

On surveying the ancient Indian literature, detailed description of fundamental principles for treatment of children are found. These fundamentals are guidelines to a physician, for treating the children.

Caraka[2] has advocated that the physician should immediately start the treatment of a child as soon as, very early features of the desease are detected. Before starting the treatment, following facts should be kept in mind:

1. Nature of child and disease
2. Etiological factors
3. Prodromal signs/symptoms of disease
4. Sign/symptoms of disease, and
5. Upaśaya of disease.

Besides observing the above factors, the child should be examined very thoroughly. After having final diagnosis, treatment should be started. For examination of sick child, Kaśyapa[3] has added few more points:

(i) The ill child should be examined very keenly, to draw inference by their activities, related to the disease.

(ii) The examination must be thorough and should be performed daily.

The above facts, established by Kaśyapa are very much scientific and are practised now-a-days by all modern physicians, especially by Pediatricians.

Caraka[4] and other scholars have considered that the children have similar doṣa, dūṣya and diseases to that of adults. Prescription is also somewhat similar in both the cases but doses of drugs are less in children and decided according to the age.

Pathyāpathya (Wholesome and Unwholesome)

Use of wholesome and unwholesome articles and mode of life, play an important role in diseases as well as for maintaining the health. Caraka has supported this view and mentioned that the child becomes healthy very shortly by using the appropriate drugs and wholesome diet. Once the child returns to his normal health, he should follow various rules of hygiene. For this purpose the child should be advised diet (āhāra) and daily routine (vihāra) opposite to place (deśa), time (kāla) and the nature of child itself. If any thing is uncongenial to the child, that should be stopped gradually, because the wholesome (sātmya) substances may become unwholesome (asātmya) after some times. Use of wholesome substance provide health and strength to the child.[5]

Children should be given milk with sweet articles (madhura dravyas). It should be diluted before offering to the child. The articles which are much snigdha (unctuous), rūkṣa (dry), uṣṇa (hot) and amla (sour) in property; of Kaṭu Vipāka and other heavy (guru) articles (drugs, drinks and food), should be avoided.[6] Vangasena has also prescribed to give milk to the ill child. He opines that when all types of food are restricted to the child then also, the physician should never advise to stop breast milk. In inadequacy of breast milk, goat's milk or any other milk, having same properties should be prescribed.

The above description have inference that for speedy recovery adequate nutrition should be maintained during the course of illness.

Mode of Treatment

The mode of therapy may change according to nature and type of diseases. Caraka,[7] the pioneer physician of ancient period, has described three types of treatments, viz., Daivavypāṣraya, Yukti-vyapāṣraya; and Satvāvajaya.

1. *Daiva-vyapāṣraya Chikitsā* (*Divine therapy*)—This therapy is done by the use of Mantras (incantations), auṣadha (sacred herbs), maṇidhārṇa (precious gems), mangala karma (propitiatory rites) including—bali (sacrifice) and homa (offerings), niyama (vows), prāyaścita (ceremonial penitence), upvāsa (fasts), etc. It should be advised in the conditions where actual relation of doṣas and dūṣyas are not established.

Kaśyapa[8] has described this therapy as "bheṣaja" in treating various disorders of children.

2. *Yukti-vyapāśraya (Rational therapy)*—It includes the use of various preparations of drugs, āhāra (wholesome diet) and vihāra (mode of life). This therapy was very common among other scholars. Kaśyapa has described it as "Auṣadha Cikitsā".[9]

3. *Satvāvajaya (Psychological therapy)*—The term "Satvāvajaya" implies the therapy for psychological disturbances. This is secured best, by restraining the mind from desire for unwholesome object and the cultivation of jñāna, vijñāna, courage, memory and samadhi.[10]

Vāgbhaṭa[11] has divided all the processes of treatment under Apatarpaṇa and Santarpaṇa. The Apatarpaṇa may be again subdivided into Saṃśodhana and Saṃśamana therapy.

(i) *Sodhana therapy*—Various acts and drugs used for elimination of doṣas come under Śodhana therapy. The processes of this therapy are known as Pañca-Karma which include vamana, virecana, āsthapana (anuvāsana), śirovirecana and raktamokṣaṇa.

(ii) *Samana therapy*—The main object of this therapy is to keep the doṣas in balanced state. It includes pācana, dīpana, kṣudhā, tṛsā, vyāyāma, ātapa and māruta.

All these above mentioned therapies may be used for treatment of children but these have their limitations. Therefore selection of therapy for children should be done very carefully and must be applied where indicated.

Various indications, contraindications, use of drugs and process for the treatment of children, are discussed hereunder as Śodhana and Śamana therapy.

(A) Śamana Therapy (Fundamentals of Drug Therapy in Children)

The most important aspect in the treatment of children is proper selection of drugs and calculation of doses. It is clear from previous description of fundamentals of treatment of children, as there is no specific difference between the treatment of children and adults except quantity of drugs, which must be less in chidlren.[12] Ancient Āyurvedic texts have ample references of the subject.

Caraka has mentioned the reasons for specific doses of drugs for children. Children are tender in nature, unable to express or mention their problems and are dependent on others. He further described the qualities of drugs, used for children. The drugs must be sweet (madhura), astringent (kaṣāya), easily soluble in milk and easy in digestion and assimilation. Drugs and foods, which are very fatty, dry, hot, sour and heavy should be avoided.[13]

Suśruta has described the mode of administration and method of calculation of doses of drugs. The child receiving only milk in diet (kṣīrāda) should be given mild drugs which subside kapha and meda. For treatment of child, when drug is prescribed to mother/wet-nurse, it should be given alone, not with ghṛta or milk. In children, receiving milk and cereals in diet (kṣīrānnāda), the drug should be administered to both child and mother; but in case where child receives mostly cereals in diet (annāda), the drug should be administered only to the child.[14]

Suśruta has advocated an another method of drug administration. The selected drug is pasted on the breast of mother or wet-nurse and child is allowed to suck. By this method the child ingest drug along with breast-milk.[15]

Methods for calculating the doses of drugs should be as follows:[16]

1. Breast fed (kṣīrāda) or a baby older than one month should given the drugs in doses of one pinch.
2. The kṣīrānnāda should be administered the drug in doses equal to the size of stone of plum fruit (Kolāṣthi).
3. Annāda child is to be given the drugs in the quantity equal to the size of plum fruit (Kola).

In annāda children, drug should be administered along with food. By this way physician can maintain the strength and agni (metabolism) of child.[17]

Table 7: Dosage schedule prescribed by Suśruta

Stages of Childhood Age	*To whom, drug should be administered*	*Doses of drugs*
1. Kṣīrāda (upto 1 yr.)	Child + Dhātrī	Amount held on terminal phalanx of index finger
2. Kṣīrānnāda (1-2 yrs.)	Child + Dhātrī	Equal to stone of plum fruit (Kolāsthi)
3. Annāda (>2 yrs.)	Child	Equal to plum fruit (Kola)

The main treatise devoted to the subject (Kaumārbhṛtya) is Kaśyapa Saṃhitā. This text contains very detailed and scientific description of fundamentals of drug therapy.[18] Kaśyapa has decided various criteria for calculation of doses of drugs. He has also described doses of different recipes like cūrṇa (powders), kwāth (decoction), sneha (oleation), etc. Details of the above are as follows:

Calculation of doses according to age of child (Kaśyapa)

1. Newborn babies should be provided ghṛta in doses equal to stone of a small plum (Kolāsthi). Upto the age of 5 or 10 days it should be slightly more than of newborn's dose. After this period and upto 20 days of life, its quantity should be equal to that of half plum fruit.
2. Dose should be equal to one Kola at the age of 1 month, somewhat more at 2 months of age and equal to 2 Kola at the age of 3 months.

3. In 4th month, the dose should be equal to a dry āmalaka but should be equal to a wet (fresh) āmalaka at the age of 5th and 6th month. However, in 7th and 8th month, it should be slightly more than a wet (fresh) āmalaka.

The dose of herbal medicines should be equal to one quarter of the dose of ghṛta, upto the age of 8th month. After this age, the drug should be prescribed after dissolving in water.[19]

At another place Kaśyapa has advocated the amount of drug equal to viḍanga phala in case of newborn. At this age, the drug should be administered with madhu (honey) and ghṛta. The doses should be increased simultaneously with the age of the child, but in any case it should not exceed the quantity equal to a wet (fresh) āmalaka.[20]

Dosage schedule according to strength of Agni (Kaśyapa)

1. Kṣīrānnāda, with predominance of Vāta, their digestive power (agni) is not very much in balanced form. Thus, the doses of ghṛta should be adjusted according to one's own agni.
2. Digestive capacity (Jaṭharāgni) of annāda children is much more balanced than the Kṣīrānnāda. Due to this reason, the doses should be equal to an āmalaka.

Doses for these children (Kṣīrānnāda and annāda) may be increased according to age and strength of agni.[21]

Dosage schedule for different recipes[22]

(a) Doses of Cūrṇa (powders)—The dose of dīpanīya cūrṇa should be as much as can be held on the terminal phalanx of index finger and double of it in Jīvanīya and Saṃśamnīya cūrṇas, but it should be half for the cūrṇas used for emesis and purgation.

Table 8: Dosage schedule described by Kaśyapa (According to Age)

Age	*Doses*	*Remarks*
Newborn	Equal to stone of small plum fruit (Kolāsthi)	Upto the age of 8th month, drug should be prescribed with honey (madhu) and ghṛta (Sarpi)
Upto 5 or 10 days	Slightly more than above	
10 to 20 days	Equal to half plum fruit	
Upto 1 month	Equal to one plum fruit	
1-2 months	Slightly more than the dose of one month	
3rd month	Equal to two plum fruits (Kola)	
4th month	Equal to a dry Āmalaka	
5th and 6th months	Equal to wet (fresh) Āmalaka	
7th and 8th months	Slightly more than one wet Āmalaka	
1 to 16 years	According to strength of Agni	Administered, after dissolving in water

The cūrṇas, prescribed for balancing doṣas, with Śarkarā (sugar) and madhu (honey), should be given in dose of two prastha.

(b) Kvātha (decoction)—The powder of emetic and purgative kvātha should be one prastha, while it should be two prastha in case of dīpanīya and saṃśamnīya kvātha.

(c) Kalka (paste)—The dose of dīpanīya kalka is one akṣa (karṣa). It is double in Jīvanīya and Saṃśamnīya kalka but half of dīpanīya, for emetic and purgative kalkas.

(d) Sneha (Oleation)—Doses of Sneha for emetic and purgative purposes are as follows:

   i. For the purpose of śleṣmika vamana (emesis) the dose of medicated ghṛta should be given in sufficient quantity (according to agni-bala).

   ii. On vitiation of pitta, the purgation should be induced by ghṛta (medicated with purgative drugs), in the amount of half quantity to that of ghṛta (used for emesis).

   iii. In śleṣmika emesis (vamana) and purgation (virecana), the doses of ghṛta (medicated with dīpanīya, śāmaka and jīvanīya drugs) should be equal to previous one.

   The dose of Kumbhasarpi, according to the age and strength of child must be four times, one third, three fourth or half of ordinary ghṛta.

It is quite interesting to note that Kaśyapa has given an indication of toxicity of drugs, when used for long period. According to him a drug should never be used for a long period in children below the age of 12 years. If this rule is not followed, the child loses his strength and age.

Kaśyapa has mentioned an another very important point that any drug should not be suddenly discontinued even after complete cure of the disease. The dose of drug should be reduced gradually and maintenance dose be continued for some more days even after recovery.[23]

Vāgbhaṭa has followed Suśruta for describing mode of administration of drug to small children.[24]

Cakrapāṇi has simplified the calculation of doses. At the age of one month, the child should be given a drug (herbal) in the dose of one Rattī (125 mg). The dose should be increased by one rattī every month till one year of age. The drugs, upto this age are administered with madhu, breast milk, sitā (sugar-candy) or ghṛta, according to doṣas. After the age of one year, the doses should be increased one māsā (one gram) every year upto 16 years of age.[25]

Table 9: Dosage schedule of Kaśyapa (on the basis of different recipes)

Recipes	*Special indications*	*Doses*
Cūrṇa	Dīpanīya	Equal to terminal phalanx
	Jīvanīya and Saṃśamnīya	Equal to two terminal phalanx
	Vamana and virecanīya	Half of the phalanx
	Cūrṇa used in tridoṣaghna Kaṣāyas	Two prastha
Kwātha	Emetics and purgatives	One prasṛta
	Dīpanīya and Saṃśamnīya	Two prasṛta
Kalka	Dīpanīya	One akṣa
	Jīvanīya and Saṃśamnīya	Two akṣa
	Vāmaka and Virecaka	Half akṣa
Sneha	—	According to strength of agni
	Kumbha sarpi	According to age and strength (4 times a day) in dose of 1/3, 3/4 or 1/2 amount of ordinary ghṛta.

Formula for calculation of doses (based on Cakradatta)

(1) From birth to 1 year—

Dose (in Rattī) = 1 x age in month

(2) From 1 to 16 years—

Dose (in māsā) = 1 x age in years

Soḍala, the writer of Gada Nigraha has only followed his previous works and not given any specific view. In the same way Vangasena has followed Kaśyapa Saṃhitā.[26]

Although all the texts, mentioned in this chapter, have their contributions in describing the properties of drugs, mode of administration and calculation of doses. However, the contribution of Suśruta, Kaśyapa and Cakrapāṇi is more remarkable. Along with the detailed description of doses of drugs, Kaśyapa has also mentioned about toxic effect of the drugs, if used for longer period. He also advised not to discontinue any medicine just after achieving the desired effect, but it should be continued for some more days in reduced amount (maintenance dose). This description of Kaśyapa may be taken as a special contribution to the subject.

(B) Śodhana Therapy (For Elimination of Doṣas)

Pañcakarma therapy has been recognised as a specific therapeutic measure. In ancient India, this therapy was in much practice, but later on its practice has declined. Now-a-days too, it is practised in very few places of the country.

There are not much references in ancient texts, for the use of this therapy in children. It is very difficult to say that this therapy was in practice since Vedic period, however, there are few indirect references which may be considered as seed of this therapy. In Ṛg Veda,[27] a mantra has been mentioned for eradication of diseases through the route of nostrils, chin, head, ears and tongue. This may be considered as a reference for nasya or śirovirecana. In an another mantra,[28] there is prayer for removal of disease through blood vessels which probably refers towards raktamokṣaṇa. In Hiraṇya Keśī 'agni' has been considered to eradicate diseases. It is possible that agni might have been used in the sense of Swedana karma.

Vinayapiṭaka, a famous Buddhist treatise contains a story, which has description of four types of Swedana (for curing vāta disorders). Jīvaka has also treated various disorders with this therapy.

Ancient Āyurvedic texts are full of description, related to this specific therapy. The contribution of Caraka Saṃhitā, Suśruta Saṃhitā, Aṣṭānga Saṃgraha and Aṣṭānga Hṛdaya are remarkable, however, Kaśyapa Saṃhitā is the only text which has given detailed description for use of this therapy in children.

In Caraka Saṃhitā, the procedure mentioned under Pañcakarma are—Vamana, Virecana, Nirūha (Āsthāpana), Anuvāsana, and Śirovirecana (Nasya). Suśruta[29] has included Nirūha (Āsthāpana) and Anuvāsana processes under Vasti and Raktamokṣaṇa has been included as fifth process.

The description available in different Āyurvedic texts have following indications of Pañcakarma therapy.

1. Use in normal healthy individuals for maintenance of normal health.
2. To achieve maximum response of Rasāyana and Vājīkaraṇa therapy.
3. In ill persons, to relieve from disease.

It is the opinion of most of the ancient scholars that Pañcakarma therapy not be administered to children, however, it may be admissible only in emergency conditions. Kaśyapa opines that child and dhātri, both should be prescribed śodhana (Pañcakarma) therapy because vitiated doṣas come in child from dhātrī, through breast milk.[30]

(a) *Purva Karma*

The processes performed before the Pañcakarma are known as Pūrvakarma, which include Snehana and Svedana. Doṣas can not be removed completely by pañcakarma, if pūrvakarma is not performed. By performing these processes, doṣas are eliminated properly and there is no chance of recurrence. Caraka and Suśruta both have explained this concept with the example of a dry wood.[31]

(i) Snehana (Oleation Therapy)

The term 'Sneha' is derived from root 'Sniha,' means love, oil, rasa, etc. Thus, the process which produces sneha, visyandana, mṛdutā (softness) and kledana (smoothness) in the body, is called Snehana.

In children, Snehana is done mostly for increasing health and vitality. Normally, snehana is the first therapy, employed in children. In newborn, just after birth Balā-Taila is applied as massage (abhyañjana) before giving bath.[32] For Jāta-karma, the child is offered mixture of ghṛta and honey. Ghṛta has definite role in first four days feeding of newborn.[33] Later on various medicated ghṛta like Brāhmī ghṛta, Aṣṭamangala ghṛta, etc. are used. These above procedures and preparations serve the purpose of Snehana, however, some of these are used as routine while some of them are for therapeutic purpose.

Caraka opines that a small amount of sneha is very effective for children. It acts as anabolic (Bṛṃhaṇa) and also increases general vitality as well mental capacity (including memory and retention power).[34] Accoring to Suśruta[35] use of Sneha (Oleation) should be advised for children in summer season and various medicated ghṛtas are mentioned for the children of different age group, i.e. Kṣīrāda, Kṣīrānnāda and Annāda.

Kaśyapa is also of opinion that snehana should be given in very minute quantity. He has considered that ghṛta is appropriate for children, amongst various other types of sneha. However, Kaśyapa has restricted snehana in Kṣīrāda.[36] This restriction may be due to the fact that Kṣīrāda (infants) have more predominance of kapha than the children of high age group (i.e., Kṣīrānnāda and annāda). Vāgbhaṭa[37] has explained the above concept of Kaśyapa that main diet of children is milk and ghṛta. Due to consumption of this, the chidlren are of unctuous body (snigdha), therefore, snehana is not required for small children. If it become necessary then physician can induce them for mild emesis, without performing snehana.

The medicines (drugs and snehas) used for snehana are mostly applied topically. Mode of action of these are not understood very well and also about the absorption capacity of skin.

Few drugs readily penetrate the intact skin. Absorption of these drugs is proportional to the surface area over which they are applied and to their lipid solubility, since the epidermis behave as a lipid barrier. Absorption through the skin can be enhanced by suspending the drug in an oily vehicle and rubbing the resulting preparation into the skin. This method of administration is known 'inunction,' because hydrated skin is more permeable than dry skin. Infant skin is more permeable than adult skin. On looking to the concepts of modern science, it is really the matter of surprise that how the ancient scholars considered the above facts and used oily preparations for snehana so that the drugs used topically may penetrate the skin.

(ii) Svedana (Sudation)

Svedana is the process by which body sweat is expelled out. Caraka explained that this therapy removes the stiffness, heaviness and temperature of body. It is only Kaśyapa,[38] who has given extensive description of Svedana Karma, especially for children. The child suffering from rigidity (staimitya), hardness (kaṭhorata), constipation (malabandha), retention of urine/stool (ānāha), suppression of voice (vāṇī nigraha), nausea (hṛllāsa), anorexia (aruci), tympanitis (alasaka), unability to bear cold, cramps (kampana).

By observing these above features of Vātaśleṣmika or sparate vātika and śleṣmika swedana should be performd. In predominance of Vāta or Kapha, snigdha and rūkṣa svedana should be prescribed, respectively.

The following facts must be considered very carefully, before starting the therapy:

a. Age and physical condition of child.

b. Season and nature of the disease.

Nature of Svedana According to Body Parts

Kaśyapa[39] has mentioned that Svedana may be mild, moderate or strong in nature according to the body parts, exposed for therapy which is shown in the following Table 10.

Table 10: Nature of Svedana according to body parts

Type of Svedana	*Body parts*
1. Mṛdu (Mild)	Testicles, cardiac region and eyes.
2. Madhya (Moderate)	Genitals, groin region, and joints.
3. Mild, moderate or strong (Mahāsveda) according to need	All other body parts.

Care of Eyes and Cardiac Region (During Svedana of Whole Body)

The eyes should be covered very well with the leaves of Kumuda, Utpala or Kamala or by a soft cloth. During the process of Svedana various articles like pearls, candrakānta-maṇi and pots filled with cold water should be kept continuously in contact of cardiac region (Hṛdaya Pradeśa).

The purpose of this act is to provide coolness.[40] The water filled in pots may also be helpful in maintaining humidity. At the time of Svedana, mouth should remain filled with powder of Karpūra or with juice of citrus fruits mixed with unrefined sugar (Khāṇḍa) or with drākṣā for easy procedure.[41] Filling of mouth with these articles may be helpful to prevent the consequence of dehydration, i..e, dryness of mouth, etc. Due to filled mouth, the child takes breath through nostrils. The dry and warm air when goes through nostrils, gets humidified and only then reach to lung.

Types of Sveda

It is the duty of physician to select proper type/method of Svedana, according to disease and physical strength of the child. Kaśyapa has mentioned its eight types, however, other previous scholars have also mentioned about various svedas, but those are not especially mentioned for children, therefore, not mentioned here.

Types of Sveda, mentioned by Kaśyapa[42] are:

1. Hasta-Sveda
2. Pradeha
3. Nāḍi Sveda
4. Prastara Sveda
5. Saṃkara-Sveda
6. Upnāha
7. Avagāha and
8. Pariṣeka.

1. *Hasta-Sveda*

It is applicable in infants upto the age of four months. It is performed by applying warm hand of physican or attendant, over desired part of body. The hand should be warmed in smokeless flame.

2. *Pradeha*

It is effective in inflammatory conditions of throat, head, back or nape of the neck (manyā), ear, eyes, chin and chest.

Luke-warm paste preapred with Eraṇḍa, Vrsa, bark and leaf of Śigru, cow's urine, Kiṇva and Saindhava, is applied over affected area. It is changed frequently as the previous one becomes cold. Application of cow-dung may also serve the same purpose.

3. *Nāḍi Sveda*

This type of Sveda is applied with Vaṃśa, Muñja or Nala after covering the desired area with cloths.

4. *Prastara -Sveda*

For application of Prastara-Sveda, warmed Pulaka (Kṣudra dhānya) of Tuṣa, Payasa or leaves of Śweta Eraṇḍa, Rakta Eraṇḍa and Arka. After giving proper massage, the child is placed over the layer of above paste, properly covered with cloths. Warmed paste of medicine should be changed frequently, as desired.

5. *Saṃkara-Sveda*

A lump is prepared with warmed Pāyąsa, Kṛśarā (with salt and sneha), meat, three hard articles (Sikatā, pānśu and stone, as described by Caraka) with Kiṇva, Alasī, curd and milk. It is applied locally on desired body parts.

Vāgbhaṭa has described it as Piṇḍa-Sveda.

6. *Upanāha*

It is a type of poultice, prepared with Kiṇva, Alasī, curd, milk, saindhava, sour articles (Kāñjī), Kuṣṭha and sneha (Tila oil). Caraka has clarified the mode of application and mentioned that the warm mixture should bind with a piece of cloth or leather, on affected part.

7. *Avagāha*

The stanza, describing Avagāha-Sveda, is incomplete. With available description, it can be said that this sweda should be performed with the warmed Māmsa-rasa of ass, sheep, goat, cat, rat (undra), tiger, lion and bear.

Suśruta has described it as drava-sveda.

8. *Pariṣeka*

The description of Pariseka is not available in Kaśyapa Saṃhitā due to missing of some description in available original manuscript. Caraka has given the description of Pariṣeka and advised to sprinkle medicated liquid with oil, over the patient.

Kaśyapa, while describing management of complication (colicky pain) of vamana and virecana has mentioned another type of Sveda-Paṭa Sveda. It is applicable in children of more than 6 years of age,[43] and a piece of cloth is used for Swedana.

The sweating is produced by direct or reflex stimulation of the centres in the spinal cord, medulla, hypothalamus, or cerebral cortex. With rise of external or body temperature (thermal sweating) is produced in two ways—(i) by the rise of body temperature directly affecting the hypothalamic centres; and (ii) reflexly from the stimulated 'warm' nerve endings in the skin. As sweat comes from the blood, rapid sweating demands a large cutaneous blood flow, and therefore, dilation of the skin blood vessels, which occur due to application of external heat.

Effect of Sweating

(i) There is an increase in cardiac output but a decrease in diastolic pressure, since the peripheral resistance is reduced by cutaneous vasodilation.

(ii) There is initially an increase in plasma volume.

(iii) Pulse rate increases even if there is no significant pyrexia.

(iv) Muscular cramps may develop due to excessive loss of Na^+ and Cl^- from sweat.

(v) Hyperpnoea develops, the alveolar CO_2 falls and there is, consequently, an alkalaemia which is compensated for by the Kidney.

(vi) The person may become exhausted.

Kaśyapa has very well observed about side-effects of Svedana-therapy. Management mentioned for care of cardiac region, indicate that Kaśyapa has noticed the cardio-vascular changes during swedana.

PAÑCA KARMA

Indications and Contraindications of Pañcakarma Therapy in Children

Kaśyapa has mentioned various indications and contraindications of this therapy in children. Although other previous scholars have also given description of indications/contraindications but that are mainly for adults. Therefore, views of Kaśyapa are mentioned hereunder in the following Table 11.

Table 11: Indications/Contraindications of Pañcakarma in Children (Kaśyapa)

Therapy	*Indications*	*Contraindications*
1. Vamana	Kaphaja fever, kapha praseka, kaphaja hṛdroga, anorexia, tastelessness, cholera, cough, dyspnoea, pharyngitis, uvulitis or adenoitis, thyroid enlarged, diptheria, vidarika, bleeding from rectum (adhoga raktapitta), nausea, prameha, halīmaka, Graha rogas (skanda, skandāpasmāra, Pitra skanda, Naigmeṣa), Kṣīra gaurava, indigetion, and fissure, pain, loose stools, oral ingestion of poisons, etc.	For mother—during menstruation, pregnancy, less milk in her breasts, the child vomits her breast milk. For children—infants, disorders of spleen, diseases of hair, ear disorders, facial palsy, hemicrania, migraine, suffering from graha rogas (revatī, puṇḍarīka, śakunī, pūtanā, mukha maṇḍikā).
2. Virecana	Mother—having discoloured milk, oozing of milk from breasts. Children—various skin disorders, like—Vasarpa, Kuṣṭha, Świtra; bleeding piles; haemoptysis/haemetemesis; splenomegaly; Jaundice; anaemia; diabetes; cardiac problems; psychoneurotic disorders; Filaria; Worm infestation, etc.	Empty stomach, weak, obese, delicate, paralysis, thirst, dehydration, facial palsy, urustambha, Vātika Hṛdaroga, Revāti graha, inhalation of pure air (oxygen) and who has not received Snehana.

Therapy	*Indications*	*Contraindications*
3. Vasti		
a. Anuwāsana	Śoṣa, gulma, marmavāta, plīhavāta gulma, dysurea, intestinal colic, abdominal colic, Vātakuṇdal, Yoniśūla, Udāvarta, Sandhigraha, Gātraveṣṭana, Gātrabheda, etc.	Hṛdaya-graha, Śvathu, abdominal disorders, urinary problems (Prameha), diabetes, piles, fistula-in-ano, tuberculosis, eresepalis.
b. Ñirūha (Āsthāpana)	Hṛdaroga, Udāvarṭa, Vātagulma, Vātodara, Vibandha, mūtrāgraha, bastikuṇḍala, prameha, raktagulma, madhumeha, kuṣṭha, Śvitra, fistula, āpastambha.	Hṛdaya drava, weakness, diseased, loose stools with blood, psychoneurotic problems, inflammation, inadequate sleep in night.
4. Nasya	Cold, cough, respiratory disorders, śoṣa, hiccup, mukha śoṣa, galagṛha, diptheria, gala śuṇḍikā (Uvulitis/adenoids), apasmāra, thyroid enlargement, nasal polyps, conjunctivitis.	

1. Vamana (Emesis)

Vamana is the process by which doṣas are eliminated through mouth by the act of vomting.[44] It is the best treatment for Kapha disorders.[45] In human life, the first act of emesis is performed immediately after birth, for elimination of garbhodaka. Most of the scholars like Caraka,[46] Suśruta[47] and Vāgbhaṭa[48] have advised to use the mixture of ghṛta and rock salt (Saindhava), for this purpose.

It is the Kaśyapa, who has described different aspects of the therapy, applicable in children.

Various drugs used for emesis are mentioned by Caraka, Suśruta and Vāgbhaṭa. Apart from these drugs, some other drugs used as helping agents (vamnopaga) are also described. Madanaphala has been considered as a chief Vāmakadravya, by all the scholars of Āyurveda.

Kaśyapa[49] has prescribed to use few recipes to induce emesis, applicable especially in children.

1. The leaves of Kaṭphala, Nicula and Śirīṣa should be used to prepare decoction, by taking all or any available one.
2. Decoction of Grahaghni (gaura-sarṣapa), Kṛtavedha, seeds of Madana—phala, etc. are also used for the purpose.

The decoction should be neither too hot nor too cold. The emetics should be administered to children, in the morning, after cleaning the mouth.

Suśruta opines that in the diseases of children, curable with Vamana; milk, curd or takra or any Yavāgū (rice-gruel) should be administered satiated upto the throad (Ākaṇṭha) for induction of emesis.[50]

In Kaśyapa Saṃhitā, views of various scholars are mentioned, regarding application of Vamana in children[51] (Table 12).

Kaśyapa has mentioned that in newborns the dose of emetics should be one Viḍanga, which is increased by one Viḍanga every month till a maximum dose of the powder becomes equivalent to one Āmalaka.[52]

Table 12: Views of various scholars regarding Vamana (mentioned in Kaśyapa Saṃhitā)

Scholars	*Appropriate Age*	*Comments*
1. Kautsya	6 years and onwards.	Children may suffer from eye disorders, if applied below 6 years of age.
2. Vṛddha Kaśyapa	6-8 years	1. Drugs used for Vamana should be prescribed with sugar. 2. Emetics should be given in diluted form.
3. Vaideha Janaka	Infants	2-3 seeds of Apāmārga (without husk) should be administered with honey or sugar.

Vomiting is induced by physician or by mother by tickling the throat of the child by his fingers. An urge for vomiting should not be suppressed. Normally, 2-3 vomitings are appropriate for children. After emesis, the child is to be allowed to sleep in a quiet room with the head facing towards east. If emesis is not appropriate, the child should be again given a decoction of Apāmārga, Pippalī or Śirīṣa with rice to remove remaining Kapha. After emesis, exertional activities should be restricted for few hours.[53]

During vomiting, the complex series of movements occur and controlled by a vomiting centre, situated in the dorsal portion of the lateral reticular formation in the medula. Apart from the vomiting centre there is a specialized chemoreceptor trigger zone (CTZ) in the medullary surface. Most of the drugs used for emesis, actually stimulate the vomiting centre directly. Pharmacology of various Āyurvedic drugs used for emesis is not known, that how, they stimulate the vomiting.

Excessive vomiting may lead to loss of water and electrolytes. There is comparatively much loss of chloride than sodium. Therefore, quality and doses of emetics should be observed very carefully because in children the above complications may be severe and fatal.

2. Virecana (Purgation)

Virecana is the process by which, vitiated doṣas are eliminated from adhomārga (rectum). It is the specific process for elimination of pitta doṣa.[54]

Caraka opines that in children, Āragvadha should be used for purgation, due to its mild action. If the child suffering from Dāha (burning sensation) and Udāvarta (retention of the feces) marrow of Āragavadha mixed in juice of grapes or in decoction of dry grapes (Munakkā) should be given.[55]

Kaśyapa has advocated to administer, the decoction of Dantī, Śyāmā, Kampillaka, Nīlikā, Saptalā, Vacā and Visanika all or any one which is available. It should be given with cow's urine and its dose should be adjusted according to time (Kāla), strength, age and nature of the disease. It should not be too dilute, too hot or too cold. The decoction is administered with the help of a pot, shaped like Conch-shell or should be licked with butter or cream of milk.

Two, three or four motions are appropriate to eliminate the doṣas.[56]

Complications and Their Management

Kaśyapa[57] has mentioned few complications of virecana and their management, as follows:

1. If an emetic acts as a purgative or a purgative acts as an emetic, it indicates overdose of drug.

2. During purgation, if the child develop colicky pain:
   (a) Child is of < 6 years—his abdomen should be fomented with warm hands (Hasta Sveda)
   (b) Child is > 6 years—fomentation with warm cloths (Paṭa Sveda).

Causes, Manifestations and Management of Under/Over Dosage of Emetics/Purgatives in Children

Children are very much sensitive with change in dosage. Kaśyapa has very well described about various causes, manifestations and management of under/over dosage of emetics/purgatives in children.[58]

Causes

The following situations are responsible in miscalculation of doses:

1. Obese or too lean and thin patients.
2. The medicine used for the purpose is very less in quantity and too much concentrated, sweet, pungent, saltish, sour, astringent and alkaline.
3. The appearance, taste and smell of medicine is nauseating.
4. If the patient sleeps during the day or his mind is diverted in some other works during procedure.
5. Consumption of cold drinks, use of cold cloths or stay in cold environment.
6. Patient is not using shoes.
7. Natural urges are suppressed or induced.

Manifestations of Under (Hīna Yoga)/Over Dosage (Ati Yoga) of Emetics (Vāmaka Dravyas)/Purgatives (Virecana Dravyas)

Table 13: Showing manifestations of under/over dosage of emetics/purgatives

Systems involved	*Manifestations*	
	Under dosage	*Over dosage*
1. Gastro-intestinal	Distension (Ādhmāna), Constipation (Vibandha), Pain (Śūla), fissure (Parikartikā), vomiting (Vamana), dysentry (Pravāhikā), tastelessness (Mukh Vairasya), frequent spitting, dryness of palate and throat	Dryness of mouth & oesophagus, diarrhoea, (Atisāra), vomiting (Vamana) pain in colon (Pakvāśaya), pain in waist (Kati), groin (Vamkṣhaṇa) & bladder (basti) region, prolapse of rectum (Gudabhraṃśa).
2. Respiratory System	Cold (Pratiśyāya), cough (Kāsa), hiccough (Hikkā), breathlessness (Svāsa).	-
3. Cardio-vascular	Pain in cardiac region (Hṛdayopgrha)	Tachycardia (Hṛdaya kampa) and pain in cardiac region.
4. Central Nervous	Headache (Śirograha), depressed state (Viṣāda)	Depressed state (Viṣāda), delusion (Moha), impaired memory (Smṛti bhraṃśa), stiffness and cramps of neck and back (Manyāsṛya and Pārśva Kampa).
5. Others	Fever (Jvara), abnormal sṛotasas	Exhaustion (Srama), Weakness(Daurbalya), bleeding (Jīvādāna), dryness of body and hair, burning pain in penis (Meḍhū).

The child may suffer from various serious complications, if purgation is too much due to overdose or any other cause. There is loss of water so patient may develop dehydration of various degree, along with electrolyte imbalance. The features of overdosage, mentioned by Kaśyapa, support this view and vice versa.

1. Atīsāra and Pakvāśaya śūla is due to overdosage of the drug.
2. Excessive water loss—Mukhśoṣa, ṣrama
3. Electrolyte imbalance—

   Sodium depletion—Hṛdaya Kampa (Tachycardia),

   Potassium depletion—Daurabalya (weakness esp. of muscles), Viṣāda

   Magnesium depletion—Moha (delusion), Smṛti bhraṃśa (impaired memory).

General Management

1. Cold therapy: It is very effective in management of complications:
   (a) The affected child should be prescribed to take cold medicated water.
   (b) The child should be massaged with ghṛta and cold water is sprayed.
   (c) Cold paste of Kaṭphala, Padma, Yavāsa, Mocarasa, Keśara, Khasa and Mañjiṣṭhā should be applied on the body.
   (d) The child should be offered cold drinks and kept in a cold room.
2. In over dosage of emetics, the child should be offered rice water mixed with powder of skin of citrus fruits and Rasāñjana.
3. Kapittha juice with honey should be administered in small quantity.

4. Use of water (medicated with rose-apple (jambū), mango, Jalavetasa and tips of Kṣīrī vṛkṣha) boiled with milk is beneficial in over dosage of emetics.
5. Use of milk, water or rice kāñji, medicated with Moca rasa or Dhātakī flowers are effective in over dosage of emetics.

The above mentioned treatment mainly contains fluid (water and milk) including various other articles like citrus fruits, kāñjī, rice water etc. which may fulfil the requirement of fluid and electrolytes.

3. Basti (Vasti)

Basti is also written as Vasti. The term 'Vasti' has become popual after the name of the instrument used in this process. The exact meaning of the term 'Vasti' is bladder (MM Williams).[59] Another reason for naming this process as Vastikarma is due to introduction of medicines into Vasti (Urinary bladder).[60]

Generally, the term 'Vasti' has been used for all types of Vastis, i.e., nirūha, anuvāsana, uttara vasti, etc., however, Caraka has used this term 'Vasti' exclusively for niruha vasti. Vasti, described in Āyurvedic texts, is not exactly modern enemata which is used to clean the bowel and to provide nutrition (by retention enemata). Role of Vastis is entirely different. Its effect and utility depend on the drugs used for the purpose. It is an ideal therapy for treatment of Vāta disorders.

Caraka has considered that Vasti is very effective, suitable and safe therapy for children. It can also be employed where virecana is contraindicated for children. It provides strength, pleasure and softness to the body. Kaśyapa has also praised the role of Vasti in children.[61]

Modern texts have good explanation about mode of action and effectiveness of Vasti-Karma. The rectum has a rich blood and lymph supply and drugs can cross the rectal mucosa like the other lipid membranes, thus, unionized and lipid soluble substances are readily absorbed from the rectum. The portion absorbed from the upper rectal mucosa is carried by the superior haemorrhoidal vein into the portal circulation whereas that absorbed from the lower rectumenters directly into the systemic circulation via the middle and inferior haemorrhoidal veins. The advantages of this route are that gastric irritation is avoided and that by using a suitable solvent, the duration of action can be controlled. Moreover, it is often more convenient to use drugs rectally in the long term care of critically ill and premature infants.

Appropriate Age

It was the matter of great controversy in ancient period that at what age, the vasti therapy should be administered to children. Various scholars like Gārgya, Māṭhara, Ātreya, Pārāśara and Bhela have given their views in this respect and considered that it should be started at birth, 1 month, 4 months, 3 years and 6 years, respectively. Suśruta is of the opinion that Vasti-Karma should be avoided in children as for as possible, however, Kaśyapa is of the opinion that it should be started at about 1 years of age.[62]

Description of Instrument Used for Vasti

The instrument used for this purpose is made of two parts—vasti (bladder) and vasti-netra (nozzle).

(a) Vasti—Most of the Āyurvedic scholars have mentioned that Vasti should be made of bladder of old ox, buffalo, deer, pig or he-goat.

(b) Vasti-netra—It should be made of gold, silver, copper, bronze, iron, wood, horn, bamboo, etc.

The length of vasti-netra (nozzle), its inlet, outlet and circumference, etc. are mentioned in various texts, according to different age group[63] shown in the Table 14, 15 and 16.

Table 14: Size of Vasti-netra (Nozzle)

Age (in years)	*Scholars*		
	Caraka	*Suśruta*	*Vāgbhaṭa*
1-6	6 angula	6 angula	5-6 angula
7	-	-	7
8	-	8 angula	-
9	-	-	-
10	-	-	-
11	-	-	-
12	8 angula	-	8
13	-	-	-
14	-	-	-
15	-	-	-
16	10 angula	10 angula	9
17 and above	-	-	12

Table 15 : Size of Mūlabhāga (main body) and Agrabhāga (outlet) of Vasti-netra (Suśruta)[64]

Age (in yrs)	*Size of Mūlabhāga (inlet)*	*Size of Agrabhāga (outlet)*
1	The whole of the size in which the pankhanāḍī (feather) of kanka (a bird) can be introduced.	Hole of mūnga size
8	The hole of that size in which the pankhanāḍī of Śyena can be introduced.	Hole of māṣa size
16	The hole of that size in which the pankhanāḍī of Mayūra (peacock) can be introduced.	Hole of Kalāya (dry) size

Table 16 : The size of Vasti-netra, its Pariṇāh (circumference and Kārṇika (ear of instrument) as described by Suśruta.[65]

Age (years)	*Length of Vasti-netra (in angulas)*	*Pariṇāha (circumference)*	*Position of Kārṇika (ear)*
1	6	Eqivalent to Kaniṣka	After $1\frac{1}{2}$ angulas in agrabhāga
8	8	Equivalent to Anāmikā	After 2 angulas in agra-bhāga
16	10	Equivalent to Madhya anguli	After $3\frac{1}{2}$ angulas in agrabhāga

Different Preparations of Vastis

Caraka and other scholars have mentioned various preparations for vasti, however, these are of general type and can be used in patients of all age groups, but Kaśyapa has mentioned some vastis, especially formulated for children. Therefore, only these specific vastis are recapitulated here.[66]

1. Nirūha (Āsthāpana) vasti prepared with different kaṣāyas and sneha with honey, cow's urine and rock salt.
2. Śiśu-sneha vasti—Taila and ghṛta medicated with Triphalā Aśvagandhā, Bhutika, Daśamūla, Balā, Gokṣhuru, Khasa, Saindhava, Madhuyaṣṭhi, Drakṣhā, Śatapuṣpā, Māṣaparaṇī, Kapikacchu, Balā, Viḍanga, Cāngerī, etc. and drugs of jīvanīya group.

   It is effective in all disorders of children.
3. Taila and ghṛta, medicated with decoction of daśamūla drugs and cow's urine and lavaṇa (salt) is used as nirūhavasti.
4. Vasti for vātaja disorders—Vasti prepared with oil medicated with Triphalā, seeds of Madan phala

(without husk), Cucumber, Jīraka (black), Pippalī, is effective in various Vāta disorders.

5. Vasti for Pittaja disorders—Decoction of Triphalā, Sārivā, both Bṛhatīs, bark of Kuṭaja, Trāyamāṇa, Balā, Rāsanā, Guḍūcī, Nimba, Koolaka (Poṭola patra), Mahāsahā, Indrayava, Śaṭapuṣpā, Madhūka, Anśumatī, Drākṣā, Samudrāntā (Aparājitā), Netrabālā, etc. drug should be used with milk, honey and ghṛta for vasti.
6. Vasti for kaphaja disorders—Decoction of Triphalā, Devadāru, Bhūtīka, Karañja, Pūtikarañja, Citraka, Ekāṣṭhīlā (Pāṭhā), Viṣāṇī (Kṣīra kakolī), Pippalīmūla, Trivṛtta, Dantīmūla, Dravantī, etc. drugs with Saindhava, oil and cow's urine is used to prepare vasti. It should be used warm.
7. Vasti for disorders of all doṣas (Sarva doṣaghna)—Decoction of Kartṛaṇa, Khasa, Bhūtīka, Triphalā, Rāsanā, Aśvagandhā, Aśvadaṃṣṭrā, Sahijana, Trivṛtta, Śatāvarī, Elā (laghu), Punarnavā, Bhārangī, Paṭola-patra, Ajamoda, Madana phala.
8. As anuvāsana vasti, use of Phala taila, Eraṇḍa vasti,[67] etc. are mentioned in various disorders like pain in abdomen, worm infestation and pain in other body parts.

Causes and Manifestations of Under/Over Dosage of Vasti and Their Management

Kaśyapa[69] has mentioned various causes and manifestations of under/over dosage of vastis, given to children. General management is also described.

Table 17: Dosage of Auṣadha dravyas, according to age, for Vasti (Suggested by Caraka, Kaśyapa and Vāgbhaṭa)[68]

Age in Years	*Dosage Schedule*					
	Caraka		*Kaśyapa*	*(Vātsya)*	*Vāgbhaṭa*	
1	$\frac{1}{2}$ Prasṛta	40 gm	-	-	1 Pala	40 gm
2	1 ,,	80 "	3 Karṣa	30 gm	2	80 "
3	1$\frac{1}{2}$ "	120 "	-	-	3	120 "
4	2 "	160 "	1 Pala	40"	4	160 "
5	2$\frac{1}{2}$ "	200 "	-	-	5	200 "
6	3 "	240 "	1 Prastha	640 "	6	240 "
7	3$\frac{1}{2}$ "	280 "	-	-	7	280 "
8	4 "	320 "	-	-	8	320 "
9	4$\frac{1}{2}$ "	360 "	-	-	9	360 "
10	5 "	400 "	-	-	10	400 "
11	5$\frac{1}{2}$ "	440 "	-	-	11	440 "
12	6 "	480 "	2 Prashta	1280 gm	12	480 "
13	7 "	560 "	-	-	7 Prsas.	560 "
14	8 "	640 "	-	-	8 "	640 "
15	9 "	720 "	-	-	9 "	720 "
16	10 "	800 "	4 Prastha	2560 gm	10 "	800 "

The dosages described by the Caraka (also followed by Vāgbhaṭa) are seen more appropriate for the age.

Causes

(a) Under dosage of vasti—

- (i) Rectum is full of stool, gases and mucous.
- (ii) Nosel of instrument is not straight.
- (iii) Bladder of instrument is loose.
- (iv) Medicines are not pushed properly.

(b) Over dosage of Vasti—

(i) The medicine is pushed high up due to presence of different doṣas, stool and full bladder.

(ii) The child is thirsty, hungry, fatigued, having anxiety, feeling of sorrow or fear.

These above causes are also mentioned previously by Caraka.

Manifestations

In both the conditions, the child may immediately suffer from thirst, loss of consciousness, fever, nausea, burning sensation, cardiac problem and pain. Later on the child may have some complaints of piles, anaemia, jaundice.

Management

1. Snehana, Svedana, Vamana, Virecana, Āsthapāna, Phalavarti and congenial diet should be prescribed according to doṣa.
2. In the condition of under dosage, the child should be offered, the paste of Kumuda and Kuṣṭha or bile of cow with water.

   Cow's urine with Harītakī or Saindhava, Saptalā and Trivṛtta is also effective.
3. In the condition of over dosage, the child should be provided proper rest. Once he regains strength, he should be tortured (Pīḍana) and cold water should be sprinkled.
4. Use of Phalavarti : The use of Phalavarti is indicated, if the child have complaints of Ānāha or Śūla.

   These, vartis used for this purpose, are prepared with Kiṇva, Siddhārthaka, Māṣa, Saindhava, Jaggery and oil. Its shape should be like yava. In case of Ānāha 5-7 vartis are used, according to age.

5. Diet—Śāli rice and diluted mixed meat soup of Jāngala animals and birds should be offered.

4. Nasya (Śirovirecana)

The use of drugs or medicated sneha through nostrils is knowns as Nasya.[70] This therapeutic measure is specially indicated for the treatment of diseases of head.[71]

Caraka has mentioned five types of nasya in which Pratimarśa is the mildest one, therefore, it can be administered to children. In this nasya, snehas are used by nostrils and can be taken without any harm.[72] Vāgbhaṭa has also divided it into two specific types, according to doses of sneha used. These are—marśa (10 drops) and pratimarśa (2 drops) and are indicated for children.[73]

Kaśyapa has described mode of administration, dosage schedule and various types of nasyas, useful for children.[74]

Drugs given by this route are quickly absorbed and produce rapid local and systemic effect. Blood levels of volatile substances can be conveniently controlled as their absorption and excretion through the lungs are governed by the law of gases.

The drugs, used for nasya-karma should be carefully selected because after absorption, may directly go to the left side of the heart through the pulmonary veins and may produce cardiac toxicity.

Mode of Administration

Kaśyapa has mentioned the proper mode of administration of nasya in children:

1. The child should be kept in the lap of the mother and holded properly and forcefully, or the child should lie down with head slightly retracted. Area around nose should be fomented and dry powdered medicine should be inhaled or put in the nose.

2. The nasya should not be given too fast or too slow. If given fast, the child may collapse or may suffer from breathlessness, cough, hiccup, salivation and suppression of voice.
3. The medicine used for nasya should not be much concentrated or diluted and should not be much hot or cold.
4. This therapy should be administered only in emergency and should be avoided in the condition of thirst, after drinking water, cold, indigestion, vāta disorders, fever and exhaustion.

Nasya Therapy

(a) In infants—In breast fed babies and infants, Kaṭu taila and ghṛta mixed with saindhava should be used. It is dropped in the nostril with the help of fingers in dose of 2-3 drops. Nostrils should be closed for a moment.

(b) In older children—In kaphaja and vātaja disorders of head, paste of two or three of the following drugs should be prepared and mixed with lemon or ginger juice, honey, dried black grapes (drākṣā). This preparation is inhaled or put in the nostrils.

Drugs—Praśniparṇī, Pippalī, Ikṣvāku, Kṣavaka, Pravraka, seeds of Sahijana, Śirīṣa, Apāmārga, Amalatāsa and Rāsanā, Mayūraka (Apāmārga), Saindhava and Sauvarcala salt, Varānga (Amalavetasa), Dālacīnī, Jyotiṣmatī, and Viśvabheṣaja (Śuṇṭhī).

In small children, the above drugs should be used as nasal drops, after mixing in kaṭu taila, majjā or cow's urine.

Suśruta[75] and Vāgbhaṭa[76] have restricted the use of nasya in children below 7 years of age, however, Kaśyapa[77] has opinion that it may be prescribed even in breast fed babies.

5. Raktamokṣaṇa (Blood Letting)

Raktamokṣaṇa is the 5th karma of Pañcakarma mentioned by Suśruta[78] and Vāgbhaṭa,[79] however, Caraka has not included it into Pañcakarma.

The process of taking out blood from the body is known as Raktamokṣaṇa. It is performed to manage the diseases caused by rakta and pitta.[80] Various processes may be selected, according to requirements. These are Praccanna, Śirāvedha, and raktamokṣana by Jalaukā, Ṣranga, Alābū Śaṭīyantra.

Jalaukā is the mildest of all the above methods, therefore, particularly suitable for children.[81]

Jalaukā (Leech)

Suśruta has mentioned about 12 varieties of Jalaukās, six of them are poisonous and remaining six are non-poisonous.[82]

Śodhana

Before the use of Jalaukā for the process, it is purified with water, containing Haridrā and Sarṣapa, applied on leech body. These are put into the pot filled with water for 48 minutes. Vāgbhaṭa has suggested that these should be kept in Kañji or takra and washed thoroughly.

Mode of Application

The patient is asked to lie down and the desired part is rubbed with powdered cow-dung and clay, gently. The body of the leech is covered with a piece of wet cloth and then applied to the part. To fix it quickly, a drop of milk or blood is put on the part. The leech is allowed to suck impure blood. A small quantity of salt should be sprinkled on its head, to remove it from the part.[83]

After removing, the leech is kept upon powdered rice and then it is hold by the left thumb and fingers at the tail end by means of fingers of the right hand, it must be pressed lightly again and again towards the mouth end, until sucked blood is vomitted out. Then it should be put in fresh water. If it is alive and moving, then it may be used again.[84]

The leech bite is to be smeared with honey, cold water, Śatadhauta ghṛta, and astringent substances or poultice may be applied.[85] Vāgbhaṭa opines that application of leech is effective in inflammatory conditions and pruritis.[86]

Probable Mode of Action

On application of leech, when blood is sucked from the affected area, the stagnated blood is removed thus improving the blood supply of that part. The fresh blood provides more phagocytes, to ingulf the causative organisms. By this whole process, the affected part become healthy.

Modern science also advised that there are only few rare disorders like polycythemia vera, haemochromatosis in which venesection is advised.

Dhūpana (Fumigation)

The word 'dhūpa' is derived from root 'push,' means incense, perfume, aromatic vapour or smoke proceeding from gum or resin; and Dhūpana is referred for inconsing or fumigation.[87] References of this process are available in Upaniṣada, Gṛhasūtras, Yajñyavalkya Smṛti, and Mahābhārata. However, its therapeutic uses are mentioned in Āyurvedic texts. In relation to children, use of Dhūpana is mentioned very well in Kāśyapa Saṃhitā, however, his previous scholars like Caraka and Suśruta has also indicated it for children.

Caraka has advised that cloths, bed and bed-cloths of children should be fumigated with Yava, Sarṣapa, Atasī,

Hingu, Guggulu, Vacā, Coraka, Vayasthā (Brāhmī), Golomī (Śveta dūrbā), Jaṭāmānsī, Palankaṣā, Aśoka, Kaṭukī, slough of snake along with ghṛta.[88] Using this fumigation, cloths and bed of child become free from germs and insects.

Suśruta has described various dhūpa for management of graha rogas. These are not compiled here but will be discussed in the chapter of Graharogas[89] (Diseases of Children).

Kāsyapa Saṃhitā[90] contains a separate chapter "Dhūpakalpādhyāya' on this therapy and included 40 dhūpas, however, due to missing of certain ślokas, the present text contains only 31 dhūpas. Dhūpas may be of 3 types—dhūpa, anudhūpa and pratidhūpa. The articles used for this process may be of animal or vegetable origin. Kaśyapa has mentioned the process of collection of dhūpa dravyas. Along with children, these dhūpas may be introduced for dhātris with enchanting of mantra.

Dhūpas, Described in Kaśyapa Saṃhitā

Dhūpas described by Kaśyapa could be classified under various heading according to their effectiveness, like for enhancing health and vitality of infants and children, for general disorders and some for graha roga and psychosomatic disorders of children.

(a) Dhūpa for enhancing health and vitality of infants and children:

Dhūpana may be used for enhancing health and vitality of the children. The specific dhūpas performing such effect are—Kumāra dhūpa, Sirī dhūpa, etc.

(b) Dhūpa for general disorders:

Due to missing of initial ślokas of the chapter, there is incomplete description of dhūpa containing Kuṣṭha,

Pūtīka (Krañja), Ambara, Vacā, Sarṣapa, hair of he-goat and Hingu. It is effective in general disorders. Various other dhūpas also have this quality. These are—Āgneya dhūpa, Rakṣoghna dhūpa, Nandaka dhūpa, Brāhma dhūpa, Ariṣṭa dhūpa, Svāstika dhūpa, etc.

(c) Dhūpa for Graha Rogas and Psycho-neurotic disorders of children:

Kaśyapa has also described some more dhūpas which eliminates the effects of graha rogas. These are also effective in various psycho-neurotic disorders of children. Dhūpas performing such functions are—Māheśvara dhūpa, Daśāṅga dhūpa, Caturāṅgika dhūpa, Karṇa dhūpa, Siśuka dhūpa, Gaṇa dhūpa, Pañca dhūpa, etc.

Any above dhūpa is when mixed with the Daśāṅga dhūpa, then it is named as Graha dhupa, which is effective in graha rogas of children.

Articles Used as Dhūpa

Various articles used as dhūpa may be of either animal origin or of vegetative origin. These are arranged systematically hereunder. Ghṛta is used as vehicle.

(a) *Articles of animal origin*: The following parts and products of animal origin are used for preparing dhūpa:

i. Hair and skin of various animals like goat, he-goat, sheep, cow, horse, ass, coat, camel.
ii. Nails of elephant and goat.
iii. Horns of cow and sheep and tusks of elephant.
iv. Slough of snake.
v. Urine of goat, sheep, cow, dog, ass.
vi. Excreta of various animals and birds like—cat, camel, dog, monkey, cock, vulture, eagle, etc.
vii. Milk of goat.

(b) *Drugs of vegetable origin* : Mostly following drugs are used as dhūpa: Kuṣṭha, Vacā, Siddhārthaka, Sarjarasa, Haridrā, Daruharidrā, Guggulu, Hingu, Bhallātaka, Tulasī, Tagara, Khasa, Nimba, Rice, Flowers of Jasmine, Devadāru, Elā (Laghu), etc.

Most of these drugs are aromatic (having volatile oils) and some other have antiseptic properties.

Utility of Dhūpa

With the above description, it can be inferred that in ancient period dhūpana was practised for achieving following purposes:

1. Disinfection of room, clothes and bed-sheets used by children. This may help to prevent the contact of infant or child with various germs, responsible for producing diseases. Now-a-days too fumigation is considered the best method for sterilization of operation theatres and wards of hospitals.
2. Promotion of health—Dhūpana may help in maintenance and also for promotion of health. The smoke, produced during the process can prevent excessive accumulation of kapha in the body of child, due to its heating and drying effect. Since the child have predominance of kapha doṣa. Thus by use of dhūpa, kapha disorders can be prevented and child will remain healthy.
3. Treatment of various diseases—The smoke coming from dhūpana, contain various volatile substances. These reaches inside the body through nasal route, with respiration. The substances, coming by this route are quickly absorbed and produced rapid local and systemic effects. Presently used tincture benzoine inhalation is the modified way to get results of dhūpana therapy, mentioned by our ancient scholars.

The dhūma (medicated smoke) may have its action by:

i. Stimulation—It may initiate the liberation of Prostagalandins or other hormones, having response on various ailments.

ii. Absorption of drug through nasal mucosa and lung parenchyma.

It is clear from above references that ancient concept of dhūpana is still in practice, but in a modified form.

REFERENCES

1. C.S.Ci. 30.283
2. C.S.Śā. 8.65
3. A.S.Ci. Dhātrī.Ci
4. C.S.Ci. 30.282
5. C.S.Śā. 8.65
6. C.S.Ci. 30.285, 286
7. C.S.Sū. 11.54
8. K.S. Indriya. 5.4(2)
9. K.S. Indriya. 5.4(1)
10. C.S.Sū. 11.54
11. A.H. Sū. 14.4
12. C.S.Ci. 30.282
13. C.S.Ci. 30.283-286
14. S.S.Śā. 10.42
15. S.S.Śa. 10.44
16. S.S.Śā. 10.44
17. S.S.U. 64; K.S. Khil. 3.49
18. K.S.Ci. 3.115
19. K.S.Khil. 3.78-81, 86, 87
20. K.S.Sū.Lehā
21. K.S.Khil. 3.82-85
22. K.S.Khil. 3.89-100
23. K.S. Khil. 3.59,64
24. A.S.U. 2.97; A.H.U. 2.77
25. C.D. Bāla. 19-20
26. V.S.Bāla. 14-16
27. R.V.X. 16.4.1
28. R.V.X. 16.4.1
29. S.S.Sū. 13.99
30. K.S.Siddhi. 3

31. C.S.Sū. 14.5
32. S.S.Śā. 10.12
33. C.S.Śā. 8.46; S.S.Śā. 10.14; A.S.U. 1.12, 13; A.H.U. 1.12-14
34. C.S.Sū. 13.38, 43
35. S.S.Ci. 31.37
36. K.S.Sū. 22.30
37. A.S.U. 26-29
38. K.S.Sū. 23
39. K.S.Sū. 23.3-8
40. K.S.Sū. 23.10-11
41. K.S.Sū. 23.12
42. K.S.Sū. 23.25,26
43. K.S.Siddhi. 3.
44. C.S.Kalpa. 1.4
45. A.H.Sū. 1.25
46. C.S.Śā. 8.43
47. S.S.Śā. 10.12
48. A.S.U. 1.9; A.H.U. 1.10
49. K.S.Siddhi. 3
50. S.S.Ci. 33.7
51. K.S.Siddhi. 3
52. K.S.Siddhi. 3
53. K.S.Siddhi. 3
54. C.S.Sū. 25.40
55. C.S.Kalpa. 8.8
56. K.S.Siddhi. 3
57. K.S.Siddhi. 3
58. K.S.Siddhi. 3
59. M.M.William's Samskrit Eng. Dict.
60. A.H.Sū. 19.1
61 C.H.Si. 10.6,7
62. K.S.Siddhi. 1

63. C.S.Siddhi. 3.8; S.S.Ci. 35.4
64. S.S.Ci. 35.9
65. S.S. Ci. 35.7
66. K.S. Siddhi. 8
67. K.S.Khil. 8.89-103.
68. C.S. Siddhi.3. 31, 32; K.S.Khila. 8.106, 107; A.H.Sū. 19.7, 8
69. K.S.Siddhi. 7.
70. C.S.Siddhi. 1.7; S.S.Ci. 40.21
71. A.H.Śā. 20.21.
72. C.S.Śā. 9.117.
73. A.H.Sū. 20.26
74. K.S. Siddhi. 4.
75. S.S.Sū .40.26,27
76. A.H.Sū. 20.30,32
77. K.S. Siddhi. 4.
78. S.S.Sū. 14.
79. A.H.Sū.
80. A.H.Sū. 11.26
81. S.S.Sū. 13
82. S.S.Sū. 13.8
83. S.S.Sū. 13.9,20,21; A.H.Sū. 26.41,42
84. S.S.Sū. 13.22; A.H.Sū. 26.43-45.
85. S.S.Sū. 13.23; A.H.Sū. 26.47
86. A.S.U. 2.81
87. M.M.Williams Samskrit Eng.Dict.
88. C.S.Śā. 8.61
89. S.S.U. 28.6, 29.7, 30.7, 31.7, 32.7, 33.7, 34.6, 35.6, 36.7
90. K.S. Kalpa. Dhūpa.

8

Diseases of Children and Their Management

The ultimate aim of medicine is to keep the person healthy, by preventing or by treating a disease. Thus the knowledge of various disorders and related symptoms is very essential for a physician. It is also true in case of children. Scholars of ancient period were aware of this fact. They have keenly observed the problems related to children and mentioned in their texts. Vedas and other books related to religion (dharma) have not taken this aspect, except description of very few diseases including bāla-grahas, kṛimis, etc. and few drugs for treatment of some other diseases.

Probably these books were not supposed to deal with the aspect of diseases. Therefore, this job has been left upon the physicians of those days.

Caraka Saṃhitā,[1] the first authorised text of ancient Indian medicine (Āyurveda), has considered various aspects of children. In his opinion, the doṣa and dūṣya are the same, and most of the diseases are also common, except few which are exclusively found in children or their incidences are higher in this age. Therefore, Caraka gives much emphasis on bhrti, means dhāraṇa (maintenance) and poṣaṇa (nutrition). Later on Suśruta and other scholars have noticed some diseases which were very acute in nature and there was no properly known pathogenesis, i.e. Sañcaya, Prakopa and Prasara, etc., but disease exhibit with sign and symptoms in very short time. Nidāna (etiological factors) of such diseases were also not clear, thus such diseases were kept under the group of graha rogas. There were some diseases due to nutritional deficiencies named Phakka, Bāla śoṣa, Pārigarbhika etc. Diseases which were due to vitiation of mother's milk and eruption of teeth were also named or categorised. Similar patterns are seen today in most advanced texts of Pediatrics.

Almost all the diseases which affect the adults may also be in children but some of the nutritional problems are common in children, some of the genetic or chromosomal disorders are more found in this age group and few infectious disorders are exclusively of this age or their incidences are high in this age.

Modern pediatricians also given much emphasis on feeding, nutrition, growth and development, and prevention of diseases, therefore, the concepts of Caraka are not out dated but holds very logical views.

Review of all available ancient texts gives a picture that later scholars, after Agniveśa (Caraka Saṃhitā) have started adding the description of diseases specific to the children. This trend has increased with the time and scholars of later period have included mainly the recipes for treatment of diseases, providing easy and quick references to the physicians.

In this book, the references available in the ancient literature, regarding children's diseases are recapitulated and arranged systematically. Therefore, this chapter contains the description of specific diseases of childhood along with recipes for some common diseases (jvara, kāsa, śvāsa, etc.) especially formulated for children. Thus, for common diseases more emphasis have been given on the treatment aspect rather on description of disease itself.

A. DISEASES OF NEWBORN

The newborn may suffer from birth injury and other consequences of improper resuscitation. Ancient scholars have observed that commonly newborn may have ulvaka (aspiration pneumonia), Upaśīrṣaka (Cephalhaematoma/ Caput succedaneum) and complications of umbilical cord.

1. Ulvaka/(Aspiration Pneumonia)

Vāgbhaṭa[2] has first described about this disease. It is also known as Ambu-pūrṇa.

Etiopathogenesis:

During the process of resuscitation of newborn, if garbhodaka (liquor amnii) is not removed, due to improper emesis or by influence of śleṣmā (thick mucoid secretions) situated in throat, vitiates the rasa from heart, causing the obstruction of mārgas (prāṇavaha srotasas). Such newborn may present with various features.

Clinical Features:

The fists of the child get tightened and he suffers from hṛdayaroga (cardiac disorders-bradycardia), ākṣepaka (convulsions), śvāsa (dyspnoea), kāsa (cough), cardi (vomiting) and jvara (fever) etc. complications.

Ulvaka may be considered as aspiration pneumonia. During the process of delivery, infant often initiate vigorous respiratory movements in utero owing to interference with the supply of oxygen via the placenta. Under such circumstances, the infant may aspirate amniotic fluid containing such debris as vernix caseosa, epithelial cells, meconium or material from birth canal. Pathogenic bacteria may frequently accompany the aspirated material. The debries of aspirated fluid block the smallest air ways, interfere with alveolar exchange of O_2 and CO_2, which may produce respiratory distress, tachypnea, retraction, grunting and cynosis. Partial obstruction of some airways may lead to pneumothorax, pneumomediastinum or both.

Management:

1. Sṛotasas (prāṇa vaha) should be cleaned by offering goat's urine, in between breast feed and especially in the morning.
2. The ghṛta medicated with Bilvādimūla (Bṛhatpañcamūla), Brahatī, Pañcakola, Viḍanga, Saindhava, Ajājī, Cavikā, Devadāru, Hiṃsrā, Hingu, Laśuna, and Vyoṣa, etc. should be given orally.[3]
3. Milk (breask milk) medicated with paste of Trikaṭu, Harītakī, Vacā and Haridrā; should be prescribed.[4]

Contra-indications: Bath and massage are contra-indicated during the course of illness.[5]

2. Upaśīrṣaka (Caput succedaneum/Cephalhaematoma)

This disorder is also first described by Vāgbhaṭa.[6] He opines that during the process of delivery the child may be obstructed. Due to this obstruction the vāta gets vitiated and produces painless swelling on head. There is no discolouration of skin over the swelling. It appears like a second head, therefore, named as upaśīrṣaka.

Sometimes, rakta is also vitiated with vāta, thus, producing various complications like pain, fever, etc.

Vangasena[7] has also followed Vāgbhaṭa.

The features of Upaśīrṣaka, described by Vāgbhaṭa are close with two conditions—Caput succedaneum and cephalhaematoma. Its comparative description is given in Table 18.

Table 18: Comparison of features of Upaśīrṣaka with C. succedaneum and Cephalhaematoma

Cause/Clinical features	*Upaśirṣaka*	*Caput succ.*	*Cephalhaem.*
Cause:			
Birth injury	+	+	+
C. features :			
Swelling over head	+	+	+
Presence (at birth)	+	+	-
Pain	-	-	±
Discolouration	-	-	+
Complications:			
Pain	+	-	±
Fever	+	-	±

Complications like pain and fever appear due to vitiation of rakta along with vāta. In cephalhaematoma, these complications may be present when it gets infected or absorption of blood may also cause reactionary fever. However, there are no such complications in case of Caput succedaneum, while its other general features resembles with upaśīrṣaka. Therefore, it may be considered that upaśīrṣaka is the condition close to Caput succedaneum, when there is only vitiation of vāta while it may show the features of cephalhaematoma on vitiation of rakta (haemorrhage).

Treatment:

1. Use of nasya and other therapy relieving vitiation of vāta.
2. On suppuration, this should be treated like an abscess.

Modern texts are of opinion that these both conditions (Caput and cephalhaematoma) are self limiting, therefore, disappear spontaneously without any treatment. The incision and drainage is indicated only when cephalhaematoma gets infected, which is indicated in classics as the treatment like abscess.

3. Complications of Umbilical Cord

In intra-uterine life the fetus receives its nutrition through umbilical cord, which is very essential for survival. However, after birth, it becomes useless and sometimes may become source of various complications, fatal to the child. Therefore, it should be cared of, very cautiously. Improper care may develop various complications. In ancient texts, complications of umbilical cord are described very well, which are—nābhipāka, nābhi-śotha, unnata-nābhi, nābhi-tuṇḍī, delayed fall of cord and complication of nābhi due to its improper cutting.

(I) Delayed Fall of Cord

Vāgbhaṭa[8] has considered that normally the umbilical cord should fall off within 5 days. Modern paediatrician also consider that the cord usually falls after 5-10 days (depending upon weather etc. factors), but takes longer, if it is dry and shrivelled or when infected.

In this condition, Vāgbhaṭa has advocated to sprinkle cooled ash of charcoal or application of thick paste of jaggery, prepared on the ground.

(II) Nābhi-Pāka (Umbilical Sepsis)

Ancient scholars have described only treatment aspect of this condition and no features have been mentioned. Modern texts have description that in condition of umbilical sepsis (nābhi-pāka) there are presence of purulent discharge, red and inflammed peri-umbilical area and foul smell. Spread of infection along with umbilical vein may lead to pyelophlebitis with formation of micro-hepatic abscess. This may be followed by portal hypertension later in life.

Treatment:

(i) Application of oil medicated with Haridrā, Lodhra, Madhuyaṣṭhī, Priyangu and Devadāru.

(ii) The fine powder prepared with the above drugs (used for preparing oil) should be sprinkled over the wound.[9]

The above recipes have been described by Caraka. Other scholars have also found them very effective, therefore, accepted and described in their texts.[10]

The drugs used for preparing oil and powder have the properties of astringent, antiseptic, haemostatic and healing (vṛṇa ropaṇa).

(III) Nābhi-Śotha (Inflammation of Umbilical Cord)

Nābhi-śotha may be considered as initial stage of nābhi-pāka. The śotha (inflammation) may be relieved by giving sudation with heated clod of earth, after dipping it in milk.[11]

(IV) Unnata Nābhi (Umbilical Granuloma)

The umbilical stump, if appears protruded after fall of cord, then it should be considered as Unnata nābhi, which may be equated with umbilical granuloma.

The cord usually falls and raw surface is covered by a thin layer of skin. Sometime, there is improper healing and persistence of exuberant granulation tissue at the base of the umbilicus is common. The tissue is soft, vascular and granular, dull red or pink, and may have a seropurulent secretion. The treatment is cauterization with silver nitrate.

Vāgbhaṭa has also used Kṣāra, prepared with burning of pellets of goat, for cauterization of unnata-nābhi.[12]

(V) Anunnata-Nābhi (Raw Umbilicus)

The application of ghṛta medicated with powder of Aśvagandhā, Añjana, pellets of goat or sheep and Yasṭhīmadhu for proper healing of the wound, appeared after the fall of umbilical cord.[13]

(VI) Nābhi-Tuṇḍī (Umbilical Hernia)

Suśruta[14] and Vāgbhaṭa[15] are of opinion that there may be swelling of umbilical area due to vāyu which may also cause pain. They have termed it as nābhi-tuṇḍī, while Soḍala has named it tuṇḍī. It may be considered as umbilical hernia, mentioned in modern texts.

Treatment:

Oleation, sudation and unctions with the drugs, capable of suppressing vāta, should be done.

(VII) Complications due to Improper Cutting of Umbilical Cord

Caraka[16] has described that improper cutting of umbilical cord may develop following four abnormalities:

1. Uttuṇḍitā—protuberant in length and width or having broader base but less protuberance.
2. Piṇḍalikā—round and hard proturberance
3. Vināmikā—protuberant in edges and depressed in centre.
4. Vijrambhikā—having recurrence of protrusion.

Vāgbhaṭa[17] has included only two abnormalities, viz., Vināma and Vijrambhikā, while Cakrapāṇī[18] has mentioned these with the name Ahituṇḍikā. It appears that these both types of abnormalities were more common, therefore, mentioned by later texts also.

The above mentioned abnormalities may be considered as different types of umbilical hernia. When the cord has fallen off, umbilical hernia may manifest after the age of two weeks or later. These may develop due to an imperfect closure or weakness of the umbilical ring and is often associated with diastasis recti, It is soft swelling covered by skin, that protrudes during crying, coughing or straining and can be reduced easily, through the fibrous ring at the umbilicus.

Treatment:

Caraka[20] has advised that treatment of these abnormalities should be done by keeping in view the severity of the problem. The treatment should include massage, anointment, sprinklings, and use of medicated ghṛta to subside vitiated vāta and pitta. Vāgbhata has also followed this principle.

Cakrapāṇi[21] has mentioned various recipes for management of ahituṇḍikā.

1. Ahituṇḍikā may be relieved by tieing the root of Mayūra Śikhā in the neck or waist of the child, procured during moon eclipse.
2. Use of water medicated with flowers of Saptadala, Marica and Gorocana.
3. The rice cooked by the process of 'puṭa' should be used after mixing well with water.
4. All or any one of the following articles should be tied in the waist or neck of the child. These include nose of jackal, tongue of crow, umbilicus of pig, bronze, mercury, Vatsanābha or frog's bone of left leg.

Most of the modern texts are of opinion that normally umbilical hernia appears before the age of 6 months, disappear spontaneously by 1 year of age. Even large hernias (5 to 6 cm in all dimensions), have been known to disappear spontaneously by 5 or 6 years of age.

B. Abnormalities of Breast-Milk and Nutritional Disorders Due to Consumption of Vitiated Milk

(A) Abnormalities of Breast Milk and Their Management

Breast milk is the main diet of infants. Consumption of vitiated breast-milk may cause various systemic disorders along with inadequate growth and development of the child. Thus, it becomes necessary to provide pure milk to the child. Ancient scholars have stressed very much on this aspect and have given a detailed account of abnormalities of breast milk and their consequences. Such emphasis has not been given by modern scientists in this regard.

Etiopathogenesis:

Caraka and other scholars like Suśruta, Vāgbhaṭa and Mādhava, etc. have described the following etiological factors, responsible for vitiation of breast milk.[21]

(a) *Nutritional factors*:

(i) Consumption of non-congenial, unsual or unfavourable and incompatible foods and over eating.

(ii) Use of (excessive) salty, sour, hot, alkaline (Kṣāra) and humid or putrified articles.

(iii) Use of paramānna—a dish made of rice, milk and sugar boiled togethei.

(iv) Use of dishes made of jaggery, oleo, curd, abhiṣyandi (moisture producing) articles, meat of wild and aquatic animals or animals living in marshy places.

(b) *Physical factors*:

Physical disorders, awakening in the night, suppression of natural urges and attempt to excrete feces, etc. in the absence of their urge. Absence of exercise, trauma and emaciation.

(c) *Psychological factors:*

Over anxiety, anger, etc.

The doṣas get vitiated, due to above factors and move through Kṣīra-vaha-sirās (milk channels), vitiate the milk and produce 8 types of milk disorders.

Classification of Breast milk Disorders

Most of the ancient scholars have classified disorders of breast milk, according to dominance of doṣa or physical characters of milk. Caraka[22] has described 8 types of milk disorders due to vitiation of doṣas. Probably this classification of Aṣṭa-Kṣīra doṣa has been done on the basis of prominent features of responsible doṣa. Suśruta[23] has included Abhighātaja, while Vāgbhaṭa and Mādhava have added dvandvaja-stanya duṣṭi.[24] Only Kaśyapa[25] has described breast milk vitiated owing to grahas also.

Vāgbhaṭa[26] has described the treatment of 14 types of stanya (milk) vitiation—tiktānurasa, kasāyānurasa, fenil, vicchinna, plavamāna, tanu, sāndra, grathita, tāmrāvabhāsa, amlānurasa, kaṭukānurasa, bhṛśoṣṇa, lavaṇānurasa and tantumata. Hārita[27] has mentioned only 5 disorders—ghana, alpa, uṣṇa, kṣāra and amla.

Character of Breast Milk Vitiated with Various Doṣas

Character of milk, vitiated with various doṣas are described in the following[28] Table 19.

Table 19: Character of breast milk vitiated with doṣas

Properities of milk	Milk vitiated with		
	Vāta	Pitta	Kapha
1. Colour	Darkish or reddish	Bluish, yellowish or reddish tinge	Dense white
2. Taste	Sweet (madhura) with slightly astringent (Kaṣāya), or bitter (kaṭu), or tasteless	Sweet with slightly bitter, sour or pungent taste	More slightly saltish taste.

3. Smell	No Smell	Foul smelling like blood	Smell like ghṛta, oil brain or animal fat
4. Temperature	Normal, slightly cool	Warm	Cool
5. Consistency	Thin	Intermediate	Thick, sticky and fibrinous
6. Foam	Present	Absent	Absent
7. Viscidity	Less	Intermediate	High
8. Light/heavy	Light	Intermediate	Heavy
9. Water-test (pouring of milk in glass of water)	Floats	Remains at any level, produces yellow streaks in water.	Settles down
Effect on Baby:			
General effect	Slightly cooling effect	Heating effect	Cooling effect
Effect on constitution and types of disease	Vāta constitution likely to get Vātaja disorders	Pitta constitution, likely to get pittaja disease	Kapha constitution, likely to get kaphaja diseases.
General health	Thin and lean	Thin	Heavy, stout with distended abdomen.
Voice	weak, hoarse	-	-
Stools	Constipated or hunger diarrhoea	Semi-solid loose stools	Constipation
Urine	Dysurea retention of urine	-	Retention of urine

Milk vitiation with two doṣas may have the features of both the doṣas. Similarly milk vitiated with all the three doṣas together exhibits, physical characters as well as symptoms of all the doṣas. Suśruta has described that milk vitiated due to trauma causes similar symptoms as vitiated with vāta.

Milk vitiated with grahas: Kaśyapa[29] is the only physician who has described the effects of various grahas on breast milk. He opines that the grahas first affect to mother/dhātrī and vitiate her breast milk. On consuming such breast milk vitiated by grahas, may cause various complications in the child. Details are summarised in the following Table 20.

Table 20: Showing effect of breast milk vitiated with Grahas

Effect of graha	*Properties of vitiated milk*	*Effect on child*
1. Śakunī	Taste of milk become kaṭu and tikta	Kaṣāya taste—retention of urine and stool
2. Skanda	Vitiated milk shows the features of all the doṣas	Oil coloured—strong, Like colour of ghṛta, smoky—renowned
4. Pūtanā	Taste—Swādu (madhura)	Passes too much urine and stool.

Since the description of Kaśyapa Saṃhitā about milk disorder is very short, therefore, it is very difficult to give any probable interpretation. However, the description indicate that infestation of grahas may effect the child by vitiating different doṣas.

DISEASES LIKELY TO DEVELOP IN CHILDREN DUE TO VITIATED MILK

The consumption of milk, vitiated with doṣas may produce several disorders in child which are similar to the respective doṣas (Table 21-24).

Table 21: Diseases likely to develop in children due to vitiated breast milk[30]

Milk vitiated with doṣa	*Disease likely to appear*
1. Vāta vitiated milk	Flatulence, oliguria, constipation, weak cry, emaciation, suffers from suppression or retention of urine and stool.
2. Pitta vitiated milk	Excessive perspiration, diarrhoea, jaundice, feeling of excessive thirst.
3. Kapha vitiated milk	Excessive salivation, always feels sleeply, swelling of face and eyes, vomiting and other disorders of kapha along with specific disease like phakka.
4. Milk vitiated with all the three doṣas	Kṣīralasaka.

Table 22: Effect of use of breast-milk of different colours/taste, on the child[31]

Taste/colour of vitiated milk	*Effect on child*
1. Madhura rasa (sweet)	Excessive excretion of urine and feces.
2. Kaṣāya rasa (astringent)	Oliguria and constipation
3. Amlānurasa (after taste is sour)	Amlapitta (hyperacidity).
4. Kaṭukānurasa (after taste is bitter)	Vomiting diarrhoea, cough.
5. Lavaṇānurasa (after taste saltish)	Erysipelas, skin rashes, itching.

6. Tamarāvabhāsa (coppery colour)	Feeling of compression, cramps or pain in cardiac region.
7. Tantumata (having appearance like thread)	Weakness, dyspnoea and cough.
8. Bhṛśoṣṇa (very hot)	Anāmaka (Napkin rashes), burning, fever and diarrhoea.
9. Guru (heavy)	Lethargy, coryza, excessive thick nasal mucus and Kṣīrālasaka.

Table 23: Eight disorders of milk and their effects on child (as described by Caraka[32])

Milk disorders	*Vitiated doṣa*	*Effect on child*
1. Vairasya (tastelessness)	Vāta	Emaciated, delayed growth.
2. Phena Sanghāta (froathy)	-do-	Weak cry, retention or suppression of feces, urine and flatus; head disorders (of vāta) and Pīnasa (chronic rhinitis).
3. Rūkṣa (dry or non-unctuous)	-do-	Suffers from loss of energy.
4. Vaivarṇya (discoloured)	Pitta	Discolouration of body, excessive sweating and thirst, diarrhoea, body is always hot and no desire for sucking.
5. Daurgandhya (foul smelling)	-do-	Anaemia and jaundice.
6. Atisnigdha (excessive unctuous)	Kapha	Vomiting, tenesmus, excessive salivation, excessive sleep.
7. Picchila (slimy)	-do-	Excessive expectoration.
8. Guru (heavy)	-do-	Cardiac disorders and other disorders of milk.

Table 24: Five milk disorders (as described by Hārita[55])

Abnormalities of milk	*Diseases likely to appear in children*
1. Ghana (thick)	Excessive flatulence, suppression of feces, urine and flatus; dyspnoea, cough and distention of abdomen.
2. Alpa (Scanty)	Emaciation, misery, dyspnoea, diarrhoea, aphonic.
3. Uṣṇa (hot)	Fever, emaciation, growth retardation, diarrhoea with fever.
4. Kṣāra (alkaline)	Eye disorders, excessive discharge from mouth and nose, itching ulcers.
5. Amla (sour or acidic)	Not described.

These five disorders can be included under the disorders caused by doṣas. Alpa-doṣa may be considered under vātika; ghana under kaphaja; uṣṇa and amla under pittaja disorders. Though the kṣāra is the quality of vāta, however, the symptoms exhibit features of kapha, thus this may be considered as vāta-kaphaja.

Different colours and taste of milk may appear due to vitiation with various doṣas. Therefore, some scholars have described the disorders according to doṣas, while others by observing the specific features, i.e., colour and taste of the vitiated milk.

By observing the clinical manifestations, appearing in children due to consumption of vitiated milk, following interpretations may be given:

1. Milk disorders due to vitiation of vāta, indicate that there is deficiency of nutrients in milk, therefore, the child may suffer from emaciation, etc. disorders produced due to mal-nourishment.

2. Pittaja Stanya duṣṭi (milk vitiated with pitta) may occur due to having blood or pus coming due to inflammation or abscess from breast. Thus, the child may suffer from fever, etc. disorders.
3. All the milk disorders due to kapha indicates that this type of vitiated milk have relatively higher fat contents, which may cause mal-absorption syndrome, resulting in poor absorption of nutrients which may cause oedema, retardation of growth and development, especially hypoprotenemia.

Treatment of Milk Disorders

Vitiation of milk is the disorder of mother (dhātrī) but child is the sufferer due to intake of milk. Therefore, while treating the vitiated milk (dhātrī), the child should also be treated for disorders appeared. Medicines to the children are provided mainly through applying these over teats of mother's breast.

A. GENERAL PRINCIPLES

Caraka opines that for treatment of vitiated doṣa, various measures like—Vamana, virecana, āsthāpana and anuvāsana vastis should be used for dhātrī, according to predominance of doṣa, intensity of vitiation, and suitability of measures. The use of purificatory measures to the mother depends upon the severity of vitiated doṣas, i.e., drastic in excessive aggrevation and mild in slight aggrevation of doṣas.[34]

The dhātrī should be induced for emesis, after giving her snehana, she should be advised to use diet in gradual manner (Saṃsarjana-krama). After performing snehana again, virecana should be given, by giving due consideration to vitiated doṣa, kāla and bala. Samsarjana-krama is re-applied, after proper purgation.[35]

The process described by Suśruta is slightly different from Caraka. He described that on vitiation of milk, the ghṛta is given to dhātrī, followed by administration of decoction of Nimba and Māgadhikā with honey, in the evening, for emesis. The soup of mudga is offered on next day. This whole process is repeated for 3, 4 or 6 days, followed by administration of Triphalā ghṛta.[36]

Vāgbhaṭa has advised purification according to vitiation of doṣa.[37] Kaśyapa has adopted the principle described by previous scholars and opines that the milk is purified by use of decoction, emesis, purgation, congenial diet, and ghṛta—medicated with the drugs of Jīvanīya group.[38]

Emetics and Purgatives for the Use of Dhātrī

Caraka and Suśruta have described few recipes to be used as emetics and purgatives.

Emetics

1. Paste of Vacā, Priyangu, Yastyahvā, Phala Vatsaka and Sarṣapa mixed with the decoction of stem-bark of Nimba and leaves of Paṭola and Saindhava should be given for emesis.[39]
2. Decoction of stem-bark of Nimba with honey and Māgadhikā.[40]

Purgatives

1. Powder of Trivṛta or Harītakī with decoction of Triphalā.
2. Powder of Harītakī with honey or with cow's urine.[41]

General Recipes Used for Treating Milk Disorders

Caraka has mentioned a group of drugs (Stanya śodhaka), containing ten drugs, useful for purifying vitiated breast milk. These are—Pāṭhā, Mahauṣadha, Suradāru, Mūrva, Guḍūcī, Vatasakapnala, Kirātatikta, Kaṭurohiṇī and Sārivā.[42]

Various recipes have been advised by ancient scholars for management of vitiated milk. These are oral preparations and should be used by dhātri:

1. Decoction of drugs of stanya śodhaka groups (described by Caraka) should be used, except Guḍūcī.
2. The drugs which are tikta (bitter) kaṣāya (astringent) kaṭu (bitter) and madhura (sweet) in properties should be used on the basis of predominance of vitiated doṣa and period of vitiation.
3. Decoction of Sārangeṣṭā, skin part of Saptaparṇa and Aśvagandhā.
4. Decoction prepared with Rohiṇī.
5. Decoction prepared with Amṛtā, stem-bark of Saptaparṇa and Nāgara.
6. Decoction of Kirātatikta.[43]
7. Decoction of Bhārangī, Vacā, Ativiṣā, Surdāru, Pāṭhā, Mustādi group of drugs, Madhurasa and Kaṭurohiṇī.
8. Use of decoction prepared with the drugs of Āragvadhādi group. It should be taken with honey.[44]
9. Powder of Mūrvā, Vyoṣa, Varā (Triphalā), Kola, stem bark of Jambū, Dāru, Sarṣapa and Pāṭhā mixed with honey or any one of these drugs with paste of Vacā and honey.[45]
10. Use of decoction prepared with Pāṭhā, Śuṇṭhī, Amṛtā, Tiktā, Devahvā, Sārivā, Mustā, Mūrvā and Indrāyaṇa.[46]
11. Powdered Pippalī with juice of Śrangbera and leaves of Paṭola, followed by use of soup of light diet and beverages.
12. Powder or decoction of flowers of Dhātakī, Elā, Samangā, Marica, stem-bark of Jambū and Madhūka.
13. Decoction of Pāṭhā, Mahauṣadha, Dāru, Mūrvā, Mustā, Vatsaka, Sārivā, Ariṣṭā, Kaṭukī, Kairāta, Triphalā, Vacā, Guḍucī, Madhūka, Drākṣā and Daśamūla.[47]

14. Paste prepared with Pippalī, Pippalāmūla, Nāgara, Ghana vāluka, Kustumburu and Mañjiṣṭhā with milk is an effective therapy for curing milk disorders.[48]

All these above recipes contain mostly the drugs belonging to dīpanīya, rakṣoghna groups. Kaśyapa is of opinion that the recipes used for purification of breast milk, should be taken with honey or ghṛta, which is beneficial in vitiation of kapha and vāta-pitta, respectively.

B. Specific Treatment (According to Predominance of Doṣas)

Vāgbhaṭa has described the specific treatment of vitiation of milk according to predominance of doṣas.[49]

(a) Treatment of Milk Vitiated with Vāta

(i) The dhātrī having milk vitiated with vāta should use decoction of Devadāru, Saralā, Kaṭurohiṇī, Vacā, Kuṣṭha, Pāṭhā, Bhārangī, Māgadhikā, Vṛścakālī, Citraka, Ajamoda or Dīpyakā and Marica, with or without Śuṇṭhī or else decoction of Daśamūla should be given for 3 nights.

The dhātrī is oleated with the use of ghṛta, prepared with the drugs capable of suppressing the vāta, followed by use of pure wine and mild laxatives.

(ii) Oil or decoction of drugs capable of suppressing the vāta should be used for unction, anointment, massage and sudation.

(iii) The child consuming the breast milk vitiated with vāta, should be made to lick either powdered Saralā, Rāsanā, Ajamodā and Devadāru with ghṛta or ghṛta prepared with these drugs and mixed with sugar. It cures the disorders of child, produced due to the vitiated milk.

(b) Treatment of Milk Vitiated with Pitta

(i) Decoction of Amṛtā, leaves of Paṭola, Sārivā, Śatāvarī, Nimba and cow dung.

(ii) Dedoction of Triphalā, Bhūnimba, Kaṭuka and Mustā.

(iii) Decoction of Jīvaka, Ṛsabhaka, Kākoli (both), Madhūka, Kaṭphala, Karkaṭaṣrngī.

(iv) Decoction made of Paṭolādi or Padmakādi group of drugs should be used with honey.

(v) Decoction of Sārivādi of Nyagrodhādi group of drugs.

(vi) Decoction of Amṛtā, Bhīru, Paṭola, Nimba and Candana, mixed with sugar.

Dhātrī and child, both should receive above preparations to get rid of pittaja milk disorders.

Beside these above mentioned recipes dhātrī should be induced purgation with the drugs capable of suppressing pitta. Dhātrī should also be advised to use cold unctions, poultice, pouring or bathing and anointments.

(e) Treatment of Milk Vitiated with Kapha

(I) *For Child:*

(i) The child should be given ghṛta mixed with Saindhava (rock salt) and Pippalī.

(ii) The child should be induced for emesis. For this purpose paste of flowers of Madana phala and rock salt either with Pippalī or Madhūka should be introduced through applying on the teats of the wet nurse or directly on lips of the child.

(II) *For Dhātrī:*

(a) Emesis—Dhātrī should be given strong emetics followed by Saṃsarjana-Krama.

One of the following decoction should be prescribed after emesis.

(b) Decoctions of:

(i) Vṛhata pañcamūla, Ghana, Vacā and Ativiṣā or else Mustādi group of drugs.

(ii) Tagara, Suradāru, Surendrāyaṇa, Pṛthvīkā with or without Vṛścikālī.

(iii) Ativiṣā, Mustā, Ṣaḍagranthā and Pañcakola.

(iv) Āragvadhādi or Mustādi group of drugs.

(c) Dry and hot inhalation, fumigation, poultice and bath should be given.

Dhātrī should consume congenial articles.

(d) Treatment of Milk Vitiated with All the Three Doṣas

The child and dhātrī, both should be induced emesis and after saṃsarjan krama, both should be offered the decoction of Mustā, Pāṭhā, Ativiṣā, Kuṣṭha and Kaṭukī or else only wine.

Any one of the following decoction should be offered:

(i) Decoction made of Rāsnā, Ajamoda, Priyangu and Bhadradāru.

(ii) Pāṭhā, Tejovatī, Punarnavā and Vṛścikālī.

(iii) Bhūnimba, Amṛtā, Kuṭaja phala and Sārivā.

(iv) Pāthādi group of drugs.

(v) Leaves of Jambū, Āmra, Tinduka and Kapittha.

(vi) Use of pulp of Bilva, as decoction.

(vii) Decoction made of Mādrī, Pāṭhā, Tiktā and Ghana.

Treatment of Milk Disorders (On the Basis of Specific Taste, etc. Characters)

The treatment of milk disorders having specific taste, according to the predominance of doṣa has been mentioned by Vagbhaṭa.[50] In brief it is summarised in Table 25.

Congenial Diet for Dhātrī

Mother/wet nurse should consume following diet:[51]

Cereals—Śāli (rice), yava, wheat.

Pulses—Mūnga, Masūra, Kulattha.

Vegetables—Āmalaka, Brinjal, Nimba, Snake gourd, pea, onion.

Spices—Ginger, Pippalī, Saindhava (rock salt), garlic.

Wine—mild wines should be used

Table 25 : Treatment of milk disorders (on the basis of specific taste, etc. characters)

Vitiation of doṣa	*Taste & other characters of milk*	*Treatment*
Vāta	1-Tiktānurasa (bitter after taste)	Decoction of either Mudga Masan, Palāśa and both Kākolis or else, Priyangu flowers of Dhātakī, Padmaka, Devadāru with honey.
	2-Kaṣāyānurasa (astringent after taste)	Use of ghṛta mixed with Hingu and Saindhava.
	3- Phenila (froathy)	Milk and ghṛta medicated with Agnimantha or else.
	4- Vicchinna (having irregular precipitate)	Docoction of Sūpyaparṇi, Kāloki, Bṛahati and fruits of Avalaguja.
	5- Plavamāna (floating if put in water)	
Pitta	1-Tāmrāvabhāsa (coppery colour)	Decoction of Priyangu, Mustā and Sabara-lodhra.
	2- Amlānurasa (sour after taste)	Decoction of Dṛākṣā, Madhauka Payasyā and Śrīparṇī.
	3-Kaṭukānurasa (bitter after taste)	Decoction of Kākolī, Vidārī and Madhuparṇī.
	4-Ati Ūṣṇa (excessively hot)	Decoction of Candana, Utpala and Kamala
Kapha	1-Lavaṇānurasa (saltish after taste)	Decoction of Picumanda, Paṭola and drugs of Kṣīrī Vṛkṣa.
	2-Tantumata (presence of thread like structures)	Powder of Pippalī & Nāgara with honey and ghṛta.
	3-Guru (heavy)	Powder of either Pāṭhā & Vyoṣa or Pañcakola mixed with honey and ghṛta.

Table 26: Treatment of Aṣṭa Kṣīra doṣa[52]

Disorder of milk	*Treatment*	
	Oral medication	*Through ext. application on breasts*
1. Virasa (tasteless milk)	Finely powered Drākṣā Madhūka, Sārivā and Payasyā with luke—warmwater	Application of paste prepared with Pañcakola and Kulattha
2. Phenasanghāta (froathy milk)	Paste of Pāṭhā, Nāgara, Sārangesṭā & Mūrvā with luke-warm water	Paste of Yava, Godhūma and Sarṣapa.
3. Rūkṣa (dry milk)	Use of milk or ghṛta treated with Pāṭhā etc. ten milk purifying drugs.	Lukewarm paste of Jīvaka etc. drugs of Jīvanīya group and Pañcamūla
4. Vivarṇa (discoloured milk)	Use of pasted Yasṭīmadhuka, Mrdvīkā, Payasyā, Sindhuvārika with lukewarm water.	Application of Paste of Drākṣā and Madhūka
5. Daurgandhya (foul smelling milk)	(i) Use of Viṣāṇikā, Ajaṣrangī, Triphalā, Rajanī and Vacā (ii) Powered Abhayā & Vyoṣa with honey (iii) Use of congenial diet	Paste of either Sārivā, Uśira, Mañijiṣṭhā, Śleṣmātaka or Kucandana or Patra Ambu, Candana and Uśīra.
6. Atisnigdha (over unctuous milk)	Paste of Dāru, Mustā, Pāṭhā and rock salt with lukewarm water.	—
7. Picchila (slimy milk)	i) Pasted Śārangeṣṭā, Abhayā, Vacā, Mustā, Nāgara and Pāṭhā, mixed with lukewarm water. ii) Use of Takrāriṣṭa.	Paste of Vidārikanda, Bilva and Madhūka.
9. Guru (heavy milk)	Use of decoction of either Trāyamāṇā, Amṛtā, Nimba, Paṭola and Triphalā or else Pippalī mūla, Citraka	Paste of either Balā, Nāgara, Śārangeṣṭā, and Mūrvā or else Pṛsniparṇī

C. NUTRITIONAL DISORDERS AND SPECIFIC DISORDERS DUE TO VITIATED MILK

In infancy, milk (especially breast milk) is one of the most common and important constituent of diet, however, child also consumes other food articles after Annaprāśana-Saṃskāra (weaning). Growth and development is very fast in this part of life, therefore, any quantitative and/or qualitative defect in diet may cause various nutritional disorders. The main factors responsible for nutritional disorders are:

(a) Consumption of vitiated breast milk.

(b) Inadequate supply of nutrients to the child, and

(c) Diarrhoea, vomiting, etc. disorders.

Specific disorders caused due to consumption of vitiated breast milk are—Kārśya, Daurbalya, Bāla-śoṣa, Phakka (Kṣīraja), Kṣīrālasaka, etc. However, vitiated milk may also produce other diseases like Kukūṇaka and Carmadala, but these are not included here. These are discussed under the disorders of the respective systems.

Improper feeding or qualitative poor food leads to inadequate supply of nutrients to the child, which may lead to disorders like Pārigarbhika and Phakka roga (garbhaja), etc.

Śoṣa (Emaciation)

The word śoṣa is derived from root 'śush' means drying up, desiccating. The child suffering from this disease appears emaciated.[53]

Caraka has mentioned about śoṣa (emaciation) of fetus, developing in the womb.[54] But Vāgbhaṭa has given an elaborate description of bāla-śoṣa.[55]

Etiopathogenesis:

The child when sleeps excessively in day, consumes excess amount of water and milk vitiated with kapha. The kapha obstructs the channels, carrying rasa-dhātu. This may lead to emaciation of the child. Kaśyapa[56] opines that the milk vitiated with kapha is called as 'Phakka-dugdha,' and the child sucking such milk may suffer from emaciation. In its advance stage, the child become unable to walk even after one year of age, leading to Phakka roga. This infers that śoṣa (emaciation) is the initial stage of Phakka-roga.

Clinical Features:[57]

1. The child initially suffers from anorexia, cough, cold and fever.
2. Body appears emaciated.
3. Mouth and eyes appears smooth and whitish.

The features of śoṣa may be correlated with condition of PEM (Protein Energy Malnutrition), known as Marasmic-Kwashiorkar. The child appears marasmic due to wasting of sub-cutaneous fat and may be associated with anemia; various symptoms like cough, cold and fever, are due to secondary infections. Mouth and eyes appears whitish due to associated anemia. Smoothness of face may be due to protein deficiency (hypoproteinemia), therefore, the condition (śoṣa) may be considered as Marasmic-Kwashiorkar.

Treatment:

(a) *Medicines for oral use:*

1. Powder of Trikaṭu, Mañjiṣṭhā, Pāṭhā, Girikadamba and rock salt should be given with ghṛta and honey.
2. Powder of Kuṭakī, Pañcakola or Badara, flowers of Dhātakī and Āmalaka with ghṛta.
3. Madhuyaṣṭhī or both Vārtākīs, mixed with juice of horse-dung and honey.
4. Powder of Mustā, Trikaṭu, Pāṭhā, Mūrvā, Śatāwarī, Vidārī, Pṛśnaparṇī with honey.

5. Ghṛta medicated with Śālaparṇī, Devadāru, Trikaṭu, Śweta and rakta Punarnavā, should be given with honey.
6. Ghṛta medicated with Madhuyaṣṭhī, Pippalī, Lodhra, Padmākha, Kamala, Candana, Tāliśa and Sārivā.
7. Ghṛta medicated with Rāsnā, Madhūlikā, Bhārangī, Pippalī, Devadāru, Aśvagandhā, Kākoli, Kṣīrakākolī, Srangī, Ṛsabhaka, Jīvaka, Mudgaparṇī, Viḍanga and head of rabbit.
8. Ghṛta medicated with Kaṭeri, Aśvagandhā, Tulasī and Pippalī, clears the obstructed channels.[58]
9. Milk of goat with sugar-candy (miṣrī).[59]

(b) *Massage*—The oil medicated with Vacā, Āmalakī, Tagara, Harītakī and Coraka alongwith urine of he-goat and wine; should be used for massage of child suffering śoṣa.

(c) *Anointment*—The paste prepared with Balā, Atibalā, Tumbarū, Śalī, Vacā, Girikadamba in wine should be anointed on wasted legs of the child.

(d) *Bath*—The water medicated with paste prepared with leaves of Siṃghskandī, Siṃhavallī, Karamardī and Gokṣuru should be used for giving bath.[60]

Soḍala[61] has included all above recipes, which are mentioned by Vāgbhaṭa, and no special contribution has been made by him.

The above recipes contain the drugs, which are helpful in increasing appetite and tone up digestive power. They act as anabolics and some other like ghṛta provide energy.

Daurbalya (Weakness)

This disorder is not described as a separate disease, in any text, however, Caraka and Vāgbhaṭa have mentioned it as a complication of vitiated milk. Caraka opines that when a child consume breast milk, vitiated with Vāta, his growth is retarded. By continuous use of such milk, the child becomes weak.[62]

Vāgbhaṭa has difference of opinion from Caraka, as he is of opinion that daurbalya is caused due to consuming of kapha vitiated (Tantumata) breast milk, by the child.[63]

Daurbalya may be considered as a very initial symptom of malnutrition.

Treatment:

Since daurbalya is caused due to consumption of vitiated breast milk, therefore, dhātrī and child, both should be treated.

(a) *Dhātrī:*

1. Decoction of Drākṣā, Madhuyaṣṭhī, Anantamūla, Kṣīravidārī.
2. External application of paste, prepared with Pañcakola and Kulattha should be done on breasts. It should be washed out after drying, followed by expression of breast milk.[64]
3. Powdered Pippalī and Śuṇṭhī should be administered to dhātri to treat tantumata-milk disorder caused by vitiation of Kapha.[65]

(b) *Child:*

The child should be offered the meat of Baṭera, purified with other substances except fat and salts. It should be given with sugar.[66]

The meat and sugar may fulfil the requirement of malnourished child, by providing him adequate amount of protein, carbohydrate, etc. Administration of excess fat may have been restricted due to weak digestive capacity of the child. Even if fat is provided then it may fulfil the requirement of calories but there will be deficiency of carbohydrate and protein (due to comparatively less consumption of protein and carbohydrate).

Kṣīrālasaka

Kṣīrālasaka, described by Vāgbhaṭa is a type of alasaka, produced due to consumption of dusṭa-kṣīra (vitiated milk). It is also known as 'Atyaya.'[67]

The term 'Kṣīrālasaka' is made of two words—Kṣīra and alasaka. Thus, alasaka produced by consumption of vitiated milk is considered as Kṣīrālasaka. Caraka[68] has considered that alasaka is a condition produced due to āma doṣa. The āma is supposed to be very toxic, therefore, named as 'āma-viṣa.' Various features produced are due to its effect.

Kṣīrālasaka appears to be a combined form of visūcikā and alasaka and may be considered as acute gastroenteritis or infective diarrhoea.

Vāgbhaṭa[69] opines that the main cause of Kṣīrālasaka is prolonged consumption of breast milk vitiated from all the three doṣas.

Clinical Features:[70]

1. The child passes stools which are loose, watery with undigested food, foul-smelling and of different colours.
2. Urine is yellowish or whitish and concentrated.
3. Vomiting and fever.
4. Child feels excessive thirst.
5. Other symptoms include loss of taste, retching, yawning, bodyache, tossing of limbs, restlessness, tremors, giddiness, rhinitis, conjunctivitis, stomatitis and similar other diseases may appear.

All these features of Kṣīrālasaka are very much close to acute gastroenteritis with associated dehydration and electrolyte imbalance.

Prognosis:

Vāgbhaṭa is of opinion that this disease is very difficult to treat.[71]

Treatment:

Caraka opines that emesis should be induced by offering lukewarm water with rock-salt, to eliminate āma viṣa.[72]

Vāgbhaṭa has prescribed to induce emesis very urgently, in both dhātrī (mother/wet-nurse) and child.[73] The drugs of Vacādi group should be used for this purpose.[74]

After emesis, one of the following decoction should be prescribed:

(i) Decoction of Mustā, Pāṭhā, Atīsa, Kuṣṭha and Kuṭakī.

(ii) Decoction of Rāsnā, Priyangu, Ajamoda, Devadāru.

(iii) Decoction of Pāṭhā, Tejabalā, Punarnavā, Vṛścikālī.

(iv) Decoction of Cirāyatā, Gudūcī, Indrayava, Anantamūla.

(v) Decoction of drugs of Vacādi, Haridrādi or Pāṭhādi group.

(vi) Decoction of Jambu, Āmra, Tinduka and leaves of Kapittha.

(vii) Decoction of Bilva.

Treatment of various associated features like vomiting, thirst, etc. have also been described in Yogaratna Samuccaya.[75]

Pārigarbhika (Paribhava)

Though this disease has been described by Vāgbhaṭa, but followed by many others. Vāgbhaṭa is of opinion that a women, whose child is on her breasts, when becomes again pregnant, her sucking child may suffer from this disorder. It may be considered as an early stage of phakka (garbhaja).[76]

Early childhood period is a very crucial period for growth and development, because the child attains its maximum growth during this period. Due to this highest rate of growth, the child requires sufficient amount of nutrients.

Vāgbhaṭa and others discussed well about the consequences of the problem and mentioned that the infant which is surviving on breasts of a pregnant women, may suffer from mal-nutrition and its consequences like wasting, cough, vomiting, decreased digestive and metabolic power, anorexia, enlargement of abdomen and some mental symptoms, like confusion, etc.[77]

Modern concepts favour the views of Vāgbhaṭa. During pregnancy, probable factors responsible for qualitative and quantitative deficient breast milk may be physiological as well as psychological. In pregnancy, most of the nutrients are utilised for formation and growth of fetus; thus the milk supplied by such women, during pregnancy, may have comparatively low concentration of macro and micro-nutrients. An other aspect is the psychological divergence of pregnant mother from his child, to the fetus growing in her womb.

Deficiency of nutrients especially of protein along with energy may lead to wasting of body. Low resistance power may be the cause of secondary infection presenting with various symptoms like fever, cough, diarrhoea, vomiting, etc. Anorexia, improper digestion and metabolism (mandāgni) may be due to deficiency of enzymes and hormones, which are not properly secreted because these are formed by the protein, which is deficient in the case of Pārigarbhika.

Treatment:

In this disorder, the functions of 'Agni' are diminished, therefore, the main object of therapy should be to keep the agni in normal state. Other associated complications should be treated accordingly.[78]

1. The associated cough, etc. disorders should be treated by providing ghṛta medicated with Pippalī, Pippalīmūla,

Kuṭakī, Devadāru, Svarjikā kṣāra, Yavakṣāra, Viḍa salt, Ajājī, Bilva, Citraka, Ajamoda along with curd, Kañjī and Surāmaṇḍa.

This therapy is also effective in associated diarrhoea.[79]

2. Excessive hunger may be relieved by prescribing one of the following recipes:
   (i) Powder of Vidārī, Yava, Godhūma, Pippalī with ghṛta; alongwith milk sweetened with honey and sugar.
   (ii) Goat milk, medicated with marrow of Vibhītaka, Kākolī, Kṣīrakākolī, Madhuyaṣṭhī and Moraṭha.
   (iii) Ekṣuka-bīja coocked in goat's milk.
3. Ghṛta medicated with Balā, Vidārī, Trikaṭu, Kuṣṭha, Khasa, Kucandana; is effective in treating Pārigarbhika.[80]
4. Bath—Various types of bath have been advocated for management of this disorder:
   (i) Water medicated with rotos of Kṣīrī vṛkṣa.
   (ii) Bath with juice of dung should be performed in any sacred place.

Phakka

It is only Kaśyapa, who has observed the mile stones, especially period of walking. By the available description, it is clear that he has considered that at the age of one year, child should be able to walk. If it is delayed, then it should be considered abnormal and the stage should be known as 'Phakka.'[81]

Factors responsible for delayed walking may be due to inadequate supply of nutrients or secondary due to debilitating disease. By observing these factors, Kaśyapa has classified Phakka into 3 categories.

CLASSIFICATION

1. Kṣīraja
2. Garbhaja
3. Vyādhija

1. Kṣīraja Phakka

The breast milk, vitiated with kapha doṣa is considered the cause. The mother having milk, especially vitiated with śleṣmā is known as 'Phakka dugdhā'.

On consuming such type of vitiated milk, the child initially suffers from many diseases, later on develops 'Phakka' condition due to emaciation. While on consumption of milk vitiated with pitta, vāta or by all the three doṣas (tridoṣya), or his mother has various children; the child may suffer from disability to walk along with features of mental retardation (Jaḍatā and mūkatā). In view of modern science these features may be present in the infant due to degenerative changes in the brain due to malnutrition. Similar condition may take place after prolonged use of vitiated milk, which may finally lead phakkatwa and all the symptoms may appear in child.

Hytten's (1954) report favours the view of Kaśyapa that the child of a mother, having many children, is more prone to develop phakka roga. It has been claimed by him that olderly mothers are less likely to breast feed successfully. It is also true that the infants of older multiparous mothers of poor societies are often at a nutritional disadvantage. This may cause these mothers more likely to be malnourished. In these mothers milk yield were also reported less in comparison to younger women having less children.

2. Garbhaja Phakka

The mother of child (who is on her breast) when becomes pregnant, her breast milk is reduced in quantity and very shortly she becomes unable to feed her infant, adequately.

The child upto the age of 1 year is said 'Kṣīrapa.' The main diet of children, belonging to this age group, is milk, usually supplied by the mother through her breast. Therefore, in deficiency of breast milk, the child may suffer from malnutrition, due to inadequate feeding and poor supply of nutrients. Thus that child may become a victim of Phakka.

Pārigarbhika may be considered as an early stage of garbhaja-phakka.

3. Vyādhija Phakka

The child when not cared properly, may suffer from various diseases like fever, etc. Prolonged suffering results in malnutrition and may be presented with the following features:

1. Loss of flesh, strength and lusture.
2. Buttocks, arms and thighs becomes lean.
3. The abdomen and head looks relatively bigger, due to emaciation of other body parts.
4. The eyes appears yellowish, probably due to anemia.
5. External appearance of the body presents like a skeleton.
6. Lower body parts (buttocks and legs) become weak, resulting in slow and feeble movement. Therefore, he use to walk with the help of hands and knees.
7. Activities of the child become dull, thus he may be manifested with flies and worm infestations, resulting into serious diseases leading to death.
8. The hair, nails are also enlarged, appear dry, hrsṭa and stabdha.
9. The child appears very foul smelling due to dirtiness.
10. The child looks very irritable.

11. Pattern of respiration is changed.
12. Child passes excessive urine and stool.
13. Nasal secretions are increased.

These above features resembles with marasmus. However, in both these conditions (Vyādhija phakka and marasmus), the primary etiological factors are different. In vyādhija phakka, the child initially suffers from any debilitating disease which later on lead to malnutrition (PEM). PEM is the clinical condition, presented due to less supply of protein and energy to the body and may be as later condition of Vyādhija phakka. The comparison between these two conditions is shown in the following Table 27.

Table 27: Comparison between clinical features of Vyādhija Phakka, Protein Energy Malnutrition (PEM) and Rickets

Clinical features	*Vyādhija Phakka*	*PEM* *Marasmus*	*Kwashiorkar*	*Rickets*
1. Irritability	+	+	-	-
2. Loss of subcutaneous fat	+	+	-	-
3. Muscle wasting	+	+	-	-
4. Distended abdomen	+	+	-	-
5. Hair & nail changes	+	+	+	-
6. Other associated features like—anemia, infection, etc.	+	+	+	-

The above table clearly shows that the child suffering from Vyādhija Phakka may have the features of marasmic-kwashiokar. Thus it may be considered as a syndrome of malnutrition.

In reference to Phakka roga, Kaśyapa has given few more explanations regarding pathogenesis of some disorders like excessive passing of urine and stool and appearance of certain mental features related to dysfunctions like deafness, dumbness, etc.

The child suffering from Phakka uses to eat more (to replace their losses) but due to weak digestive capacity (mandāgni), the body is unable to digest and assimilate it, therefore, the child passes it with water, in great quantity, as urine and stool.

All the activities of the body, like hearing and walking are controlled by centres in the brain, known as indriyas. They are divided into sensory and motor centres, known as Gyanendriya and Karmendriya, respectively. The motor centres include centres controlling all the body movements as well as speech centre (Vāgindriya). Damage to the motor centres is an important cause of late walking (Phakka). If the hearing and speech centres are also simultaneously affected, the child become deaf and dumb and starts walking late.

There is little confusion between the scholars of today because some of them are of view that Phakka should be considered as a rickets. The Table 27 gives a clear picture. It will be appropriate here, to clarify about the confusion, that Phakka has been considered as ricket.

It appears, that scholars are probably confused with two features—unability to walk upto 1 year, and appearance of enlarged head (correlated with bossing). But on analysing the facts carefully, the whole concept becomes clear. In the pathogenesis of Phakka, Kaśyapa very clearly says that due to various causes, the child (in his infancy), become emaciated, followed by delayed walking. While in case of rickets, though there may be some difficulty in walking, but there is no generalised emaciation of body, which is the primary feature of Phakka roga. Appearance of enlarged head is not due to bossing (as in ricket) but it is a normal appearance of a emaciated child, that his head appears enlarged in comparison to other body parts.

Management

The following line of management should be followed for management of Phakka.

1. Snehana and Śodhana—The child is oleated by prescribing him Kalyāṇa ghṛta, Satapala ghṛta, or Amṛta ghṛta for 7 days.

   For Śodhana, milk treated with Trivṛtta is given. Brāhmī ghṛta should be prescribed after above processes.
2. Milk medicated with Rāsnā, Madhuyaṣṭhī, Punarnavā, Ekaparṇī, Eraṇḍa, Satapuṣpā, Drākṣhā, Pīlu, Trivṛtta, etc. drugs.
3. Ghṛta, oil, soup and meat-juice, medicated with Rāsnā, honey, etc. should be given two times a day.
4. If the causative factor is predominance of Kapha, cow's urine should be prescribed.

The above recipes contain mik, ghṛta, oil, meat-juice along with various drugs. These preparations supply various nutrients to the child. Ghṛta and oil are rich source of energy. Drugs may be helpful in improving digestive capacity and metabolic processes, including physical as well as mental tone up.

5. Physiotherapy—Kaśyapa is the first among ancient scholars, who has made the provision of physiotherapy and considered its importance in rehabilitation of a crippled child. For this purpose, following measures have been prescribed:

   (i) The child should be massaged with Rāja taila.

   (ii) Practice of walking should be started with the help of specially prepared Tricycle (Phakka ratha)—a stand with three wheels.

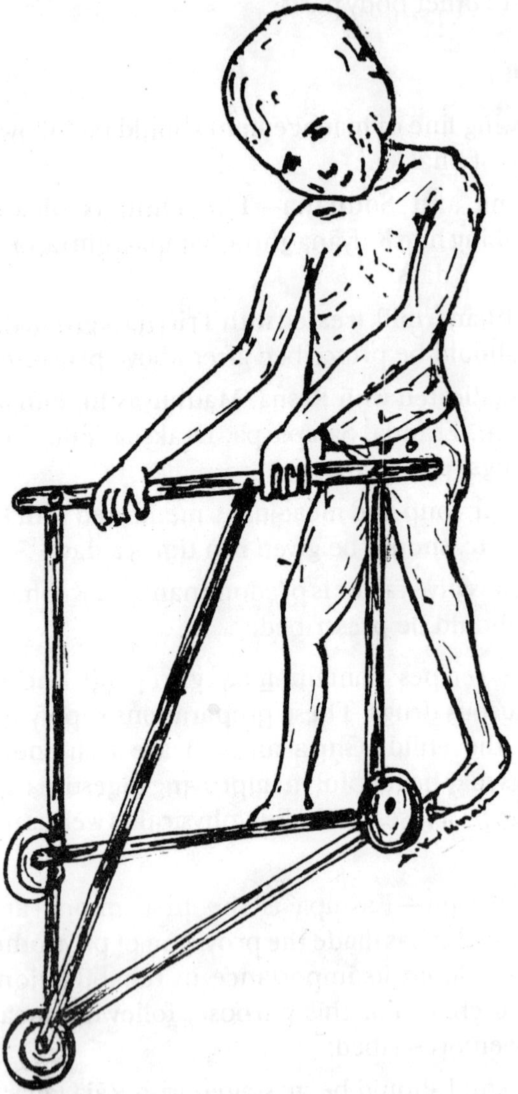

Phakka-Rath (Kaśyapa Saṃhitā)
For physiotherapy and rehabilitation of child suffering from Phakka-roga.

6. Diet (Pathyāpathya)—Supplementation of diet is an important factor in management of Phakka. The child should be offered especially meat soup, cereals (rice, etc.) and medicated milk.[82]

The above dietary regimen provides protein, carbohydrate, fat along with various vitamins and minerals, to come up from the problem.

D. DISEASES AND SYMPTOMS ASSOCIATED WITH MOUTH AND PALATE

The ancient scholars have mentioned that diseases and symptoms associated with mouth and palate, especially affecting to children are - Tālukaṇṭaka, Tālunaman, Mukha pāka, Tālu janya vraṇa, etc.

The term 'Tālu' used here refers to the palate or bregma, it should be perceived with reference to the context.

Tālukaṇṭaka

Vāgbhaṭa[83] has described that this disease is produced due to increased kapha in Tālumāṃsa with following features:

1. Depression of Tālu pradeśa.
2. Difficulty in sucking breast milk, i.e. dysphagia.
3. Loose stools.
4. Thirst.
5. Vomiting.
6. Pain in throat and eyes.
7. Difficulty in head control.

Other schoars have also mentioned these above features.[84]

Infections of mouth, throat are considered as a main cause of dysphagia (difficult sucking).

Here, the term tālu may be referred with palate and bregma both with reference to the context. Vāgbhaṭa has mentioned that the cause of disease is depression of tālu (palate). In other hand depression of tālu (ant. fontanel) is a feature of dehydration due to loose stools, vomiting, etc. which may be the associated features of this disease.

Palate forms the roof of the mouth and consists of two portions—hard palate and soft palate. Hard palate separates the oral and nasal cavities, while soft palate is suspended from the posterior border of the hard palate. Later consists of a fold of mucous membrane enclosing muscular fibres, an aponeurosis, vessels, nerves, lymphoid tissue, and mucous glands.

The palatine tonsil is a prominent mass of lymphatic tissue situated at the side of the fauces. Here with the reference of tālukaṇṭaka, these tonsils may be considered as a seat of kapha (lymph). Thus the increase of kapha in tālumāṃsa (soft palate) may be considered as tālukaṇṭaka (palatine tonsillitis).

Tālukaṇṭaka and palatine tonsillitis may be considered as same entity, which is clear from the Table 28.

Table 28: Showing comparison between tālukaṇṭaka and acute tonsillitis

Features	*Tālukaṇṭaka*	*Acute palatine Tonsillitis*	*Comments*
1. Depression of tālu pradeśa	+	+	The englarged tonsils may appear like depression of tālu (palate)
2. Difficulty in sucking breasts	+	+	
3. Pain in throat	+	+	
4. Difficulty in head control	+	+	Swelling and pain in throat due to acute

			tonsillitis, may cause difficulty in keeping the neck in the position.
5. Constitutional symptoms—thirst, vomiting, etc.	+	+	

Treatment:

1. Locally the Yavakṣāra with honey or Pippalī, Śuṇṭhī, juice of dung mixed with rock salt should be rubbed.
2. Juice of Śrangvera, Niśā and Kuṣṭha extracted with 'Puṭpāka' method; should be applied in mouth and instilled in eyes.[85]
3. Powdered Harītakī, Vacā and Kuṣṭha mixed with honey should be used with breast milk.
4. The associated thirst may be relieved by the oral use of ghṛta medicated with the drugs of Madhuraka group (Kakolyādi group). This ghṛta is also used as massage.
5. Cold water should be sprinkled over the child. This therapy has been previously mentioned by Suśruta, also.[86]

Tālupāta

It is a symptom, rather than a disease. It has been described as a feature of Tālukaṇṭaka. Suśruta opines that tālupāta is caused due to kṣaya (loss) of Mastulunga.[87]

It is also found asociated with thirst.

The word 'mastu' means curd-water. Macroscopically brain appears like a curd, therefore, ancient scholars may have considered mastulunga as cerebro-spinal fluid (CSF), because it comes from curd like brain.

Thus the Mastulunga-Kṣaya may be due to loss of water from CSF, due to dehydration. Tālupāta (depression of ant. fontanale) is a clinical feature of dehydration. Thirst remain associated with it, as a feature of mild to moderate dehydration.

It should be managed like tālukaṇṭaka.[88]

Mukha Pāka or Tālupāka

Causative factors and clinical features of it are not mentioned by ancient scholars, except few recipes. Some of the recipes commonly described by them are used for the treatment of Tālukaṇṭaka also, however, in Cikitsa Kalikā and Vaṅgasena Saṃhitā few recipes are mentioned exclusively for the treatment of Mukha-pāka, discussed while describing the treatment.

Aphthous stomatitis is the similar condition, having recurrent painful ulcers in the oral mucosa. Solitary and multiple lesions occur on the labial, buccal and lingual mucosa as well as on the sublingual, palatal and gingival mucosa. Initially the lesions are erythematous and indurated papules that erode rapidly to form sharply circumscribed, necrotic ulcers with a grey fibrinous exudate and erythematous halo. It has been attributed to a variety of causes that include food hypersensitivity, allergic or toxic drug reaction, infective agents, endocrine factors, emotional stress and trauma.

The lesion heal spontaneously in 10-14 days. A more severe form is called peradenitis apthae. The treatment consists of relief of pain by local anaesthetics and use of corticosteroids locally.

Treatment:[89]

1. Mouth wash should be done with the decoction of Sārivā, Tila, Lodhra and Madhuyaṣṭhī.

2. Local application:
   - (i) The paste prepared with the leaves and flowers of jasmine should be applied locally on the affected area of tongue.
   - (ii) Powdered marrow of mango, lauha bhasma, gairika and rasāñjana with honey.
   - (iii) Powdered stem bark and leaves of Pīpala with honey.
   - (iv) Powdered Dāruharidrā, Madhuyaṣṭhī, Harītakī, and Ajājīpatra (Teja-patra) with honey.

The above recipes contain, the drugs having properties of Vṛna-śodhana, vṛṇa ropaṇa and dāha-praśamana or these are mainly astringent, antiseptic and promote healing, besides Madhuyaṣṭhī is anabolic or Brmhaṇa, thus improvement in general health always helps in healing of any ulcer.

E. DISORDERS RELATED TO GASTRO-INTESTINAL TRACT

Disorders related to gastro-intestinal tract like, diarrhoea, dysentery, vomiting, dehydration were also prevalent in the children of ancient period. Therefore, ancient scholars have listed many recipes for curing such ailments. These disorders may manifest as a symptom of various disorders or sometimes as a separate disease entity.

Detailed accounts of diseases are not given here because these are similar to adults. Thus it has been described in very brief, however, treatment aspect has been included in detail, specifically mentioned for children.

Atisāra (Diarrhoea)

It is one of the commonest disorder of children and characterised by increased frequency of loose stools.

Etiological Factors

In Āyurvedic texts various causes for childhood diarrhoea may be recapitulated here as follows:

1. Consumption of vitiated breast milk.
2. As a complication of dentition.
3. Influence of various grahas, especially of Pitragraha, Revatī and Pūtanā.
4. Mṛttikā bhakṣaṇa (Pica).
5. As a complication of various diseases like Jvara, Śoṣa, etc.

The most common causes of diarrhoea of infancy and childhood, mentioned in modern texts are as follows:

1. Excess of sugar in infants feed.
2. Phototherapy.
3. Toddlers diarrhoea (irritable colon)
4. Psychogenic.
5. Infections:

   Virus—Human rotavirus, cytomagalo virus, etc.
   Bacteria—Shigella, Salmonella, S. typhi, E. coli, V. Cholarae, etc.
   Protozoa—Giardia lambia, E. histolytica, E.coli.
   Helminths—Ascaris, Trichuriasis, Ancylostoma.
   Mycosis—Candida albicans.
6. Mal-absorption—fat carbohydrate, protein.
7. Allergy—cow's milk, soya, etc.
8. Others—Hirschprung's disease, ulcerative colitis, immune deficiency, endocrinal diseases, etc.

Types

It may be of 6 types:[90]

1. Vātika, 2. Paittika, 3. Śleṣmika, 4. Sannipātika, 5. Śokaja, and 6. Āmaja.

Table 29 shows, characteristics of stools along with other associated features of various types of atisāras.

Table 29: Showing characteristics of stool, associated features of various types of Atisāra

Types of Atisāra	*Characteristics of stool*	*Associated features*
1. Vātika	Stool is aruṇa, phenilla, āma-rūkṣa; comes in small quantity but repeatedly with pain and sound.	Pain in abdomen
2. Paittika	Stool is pīta, nīla, rakta	Thirst, shock, burning proctitis
3. Śleṣmika	Stool is śukla, Sāndra, with kapha; foul smelling and śītala	Romaharṣa
4. Sannipātika	Stool colour is like Sneha, Māmsarasa.	-

In children, along with the above types of atisāra, two other types are also reported specifically. These are—Jvarātisāra and Raktātisāra.

(i) Jvarātisāra—It may occur due to combined effect of various factors mentioned for jvara and tendency of atisāra (diarrhoea) and in paittika diarrhoea there may be mild fever. These both conditions, when become severe may be called 'Jvarātisāra.'

All the infectious diarrhoea may have fever, thus can be included under this.

(ii) Raktātisāra—It is special condition of pittaja atisāra. The person suffering from paittika diarrhoea, when continuously consume the articles increasing pitta, may develop raktātisāra.

In newborn babies, the bleeding may be due to vit. K deficiency. If the stool is lined with blood, the source is commonly in the lower alimentary tract. When there is red blood in a baby's stool, the source may be fairly high, while red fresh blood in the stool of an older child would suggest pathology of lower bowel. These observations, however, are not entirely reliable. The commonest cause of blood in the stool is constipation, causing trauma by hard stool or dysentery.

Treatment:

Use of various decoctions and powders, etc. preparations were prescribed by ancient Āyurvedic scholars, specially for children.

(a) ***Decoction (Kwāthas)***

1. Decoction of Rodhra, Vāraṇa kaṇā (Gajapippalī) flowers of Dhātakī, Bālaka (Sugandha bālā) and Bilva should be taken with honey.[91]
2. Decoction of Bilva and Āmra with Lājā and Sugar is effective in diarrhoea and associated vomiting.[92]
3. Decoction of Mañjiṣṭhā, flowers of Dhātakī, Lodhra and Ananta-mūla with honey.[93]
4. Decoction of Paṭola-mūla, Ṣrangabera, Vacā, Viḍanga, Ajamoda and Pippalī taṇḍula.[94]
5. Decoction of Śālapaṇī, Praśniparṇī, Ghoṇta with honey.[95]
6. Decoction of Kākolī, Gaja Pippalī and Lodhra with honey.[96]

(b) *Powders (Cūrṇas)*

1. Powder of Devadāru with sugar.[97]
2. Powder of Dhānyansa, Ativiṣā, Ṣrangī, Gajapippalī with honey is effective in both diarrhoea and vomiting.[98]
3. Powder of Hṛibera mixed with sugar and honey should be given with rice water. It is effective in diarrhoea, thirst, vomiting and fever.[99]

4. Powder of Viḍanga, Sarala dhūpa, Devadāru, Paṭola-patra, Nimba, Saptaparṇa and Yavanikā, etc. with honey and ghṛta. It is effective in diarrhoea, vomiting and fever.[100]
5. Powder of Pāṭhā, Bilva, Śilājīta, stem-bark of Kuṭaja and Śālmalī with milk.[101]

Recipes for Jvaratisāra:

1. Powder of Lājā, Nilotpala, Pippalī, Madhuyaṣṭhī, Añjana and Sugar with honey; cures diarrhoea with fever.[102]
2. Powder of Lodhra, Indrāyaṇa, Dhānyaka, Dhātrī, Hrībera and Mustaka with honey.[103]
3. Decoction of flowers of Brahatī, Pippalī, Pippalīmūla with Vaṃśalocana is effective in diarrhoea with fever.[104]
4. Decoction of Haridrā, Dāruharidrā, Madhuyaṣṭhī and Indrayava.
5. Powder of Mothā, Pippalī, Atīsa, Karkaṭaśrangī with honey.

Recipes for Raktātisāra:

1. Powder of Gaja Pippalī with sugar is effective in both āmātisāra and raktātisāra.[105]
2. Decoction of Āmra, Jambū, Paṭola, Padmotpala and Śatāwarī.
3. Decoction of Pāṭhā, Toyada and Śuṇṭhi with honey.
4. Water prepared with flowers of Nārikela.[106]
5. Powder of Madhuyaṣṭhī mixed with Tila oil along with sugar-candy and honey.[107]
6. Yavāgū (rice gruel) should be prepared with moca rasa, Mañjiṣṭhā, flowers of Dhātakī and Padmakeśara.[108]
7. Powder of ripened Bilva, Aguru and Lodhra with honey.[109]

All the above recipes described for management of diarrhoea contains the drugs which are samgrāhī (mala stambhaka) while some are kṛmighna, may be useful in infective diarrhoea.

Pravāhikā (Dysentery)

Caraka and Vāgbhaṭa have not described Prawāhikā as a separate disease entity and have considered it as a special condition of Atisāra. Suśruta[110] has defined it very well and opines that vitiated vāyu initiate to move out the kapha, collected in the intestine. The person passes stools very frequently in small amount, with straining. It indicates the difference of atisāra and pravāhikā. Stool is watery in diarrhoea while it is with kapha in pravāhikā. Bhoja has named it as 'Visramsī' and Hārīta with the name of 'Nihsāraka.'

Mādhava has mentioned its four types, i.e., Vātika, paittika, śleṣmika and raktaja.

This condition is similar to dysentery.

Table 30 Showing etiological factors and features of various types of pravāhikā

Types	*Causative factors*	*Features*
1. Vātika	Consumption of rūkṣa articles	With pain
2. Paittika	Consumption of tīkṣṇa and ūṣṇa articles.	With burning
3. Śleṣmika	Snigdha articles	With ślesmā (mucus)
4. Raktaja	Tīkṣṇa and Ūṣṇa articles	With rakta (blood)

Treatment:

Mostly its treatment is described with the treatment of Atisāra.

Grahaṇī

The role of 'Agni' in the body is of supreme importance. All the physiological activities are concerned with it. Among other agnis, pācakāgni is important one, because it is responsible for providing rasa-dhātu, the basic metabolite of food and precursor of dhātus, oja and bala.[111] If the pācakāgni becomes weak, there is improper digestion of food material resulting in diarrhoea. The stool is foul smelling and may be solid, semisolid or loose. This disorder has been termed as Grahaṇī.

Treatment:

The children suffering from Grahaṇī disorder should be given following recipes, as required:

1. Powder of Marica, Śuṇṭhī and Kuṭaja should be prepared by taking these drus in ratio of 1:2:4, respectively. This should be administered in children with jaggery and takra.[112]
2. Goat's milk medicated with pulp of Bilva, Indrayava, Sugandhabālā, Mocarasa and Nāgaramothā should be prescribed for 6 days.

   Goat's milk medicated with equal quantity of powder of stem-bark of Jambū. It cures raktaja-grahaṇī.[113]
3. Goat's milk medicated with Cāngerī, Mañjiṣṭhā, Dhātakīpuṣpa, Lodhra, Kapittha, Kamala, Śuṇṭhī, Marica, Pippalī, Bilva-majjā, Nāgarmothā and rock salt.[114]

The above recipes contain the drugs which are dīpanapācana and saṃgrāhī. Dīpanīya drugs keep the pācakāgni in balance state, while samgrāhī prevents the complaint of loose stools.

Chhardi (Vomiting)

Chhardi (vomiting) is a symptom rather than a disease. Suśruta has defined chhardi as a process in which vitiated doṣa comes out through mouth after feeling of nausea.[115]

Causative Factors

Various causes like excessive consumption of liquids, fatty and saltish articles; unliked food and worm infestations, along with psychological factors also play important role.

Modern texts have mentioned following causes, responsible for vomiting in children. Most common causes are:

(i) Normal possetting.
(ii) Sucking and swallowing difficulties like congenital defects of palate, tongue, various neuro-muscular defects (cerebral palsy), infection of mouth cavity, etc.
(iii) Infections-meningitis, septicemia, etc.
(iv) Intracranial—oedema, haemorrhage, kernicterus, hypoxia.
(v) Obstructive—Oesophagus, deodenum, small intestine, vascular ring, meconium plug or ileum bezoars.

Infants

(a) *Non-organic:*

(i) Normal possetting, food coming up with wind.
(ii) Incorrect feeds, over feeding and careless handling after feed.
(iii) Migrain, allergy and oesophageal reflex.

(b) *Organic*

(i) Infections—otitis media, gastro-enteritis, whooping cough.

(ii) Intracranial.

(iii) Obstructions, etc.

After Infancy

(a) *Non-organic*

(i) Psychological-excitement, fear, anxiety, attention seeking device, insertion of finger into the throat.

(b) *Organic*

(i) Infection—especially tonsillitis or otitis media, meningitis.

(ii) Appendicitis

(iii) Intestinal obstruction.

(iv) Poisons and drugs.

Types

Mādhava has mentioned its 5 types. Out of these four are doṣika and one is āgantuja (including worm infestation).

Details of vomiting in relation to children are not described in ancient texts. Most of the time it is described to be associated with diarrhoea. The vomiting in children has been considered very serious problem, therefore, recipes to cure the problem are mentioned in ancient Āyurvedic texts.

Treatment:

The treatment of vomiting should be based upon the treatment of underlying cause. As described previously, most of the ancient scholars have considered that vomiting in most of the time remains associated with diarrhoea. Therefore, its treatment has been included with the treatment of diarrhoea. However, only few recipes are mentioned separately for managing vomiting, when it is severe.

1. Powder of Mustā, Priyangu, Sauvīrāñjana with honey and rice-water gives relief from vomiting and thirst.[116]

2. Powder of Pippalī and Marica mixed with sugar-candy and honey should be given with lemon-juice (vijaurā).[117]
3. Powder of Pippalī with five types of salts, Viḍanga and Pāribhadra with honey and ghṛta.[118]
4. Powder of Dāḍima, Pippalī, Nāgakeśara, Jīvaka and sugar with honey.
5. Powder of Āmrāsthi, Lājā and rock-salt with honey or Madhuyaṣṭhī.
6. Powder of Kuṭakī with honey.[119]
7. Powder of drugs of Cāturjāta (Dālcīnī, Elā, Teja-patra and Nāgkeśara) mixed with juice of cow's dung, should be given with honey.[120]

Dugdha-Vamana (Vomiting/Regurgitation of Milk)

It is most common in newborns and infants. The following treatment may be prescribed to manage the problem.

1. Powder of Trikaṭu drugs with honey and ghṛta.[121]
2. Fruit juice of Vārtākī (both types) mixed with powder of Pañcakola (Pippalī, Pippalāmūla, Cavya, Citraka and Nāgar) should be given with ghṛta and honey.[122]
3. Decoction of Khadira, Arjuna, Tālisa, Kuṣṭha and Candana with milk and ghṛta.[123]

Features of Dehydration and Their Management

The most common features of dehydration observed by ancient scholars are tṛṣṇā (thirst) and tālupāta (depressed anterior fontanelle). Modern physicians also consider these two features as a very useful indicator of dehydration.

Among these two, tālupāta has been discussed earlier, therefore, only tṛṣṇā will be discussed.

Tṛṣṇā (Thirst)

In case of children tṛṣṇā (thirst) has been found associated with atisāra (diarrhoea). It indicates that there is co-relation between these two conditions. In diarrhoea due to loss of water and electrolytes, features of dehydration appear. Thirst is the first feature of mild to moderate dehydration. Suśruta has considered it very fatal.[124] Therefore, tṛṣṇā may be considered as an alarming features of fatal condition (dehydration), especially in case of children.

Management

Normally the management of thirst has been mentioned along with the management of diarrhoea. However, few recipes are found in ancient classics, which may be indicated in severe cases.

1. Decoction of tender leaves of Kṣīrī, Madhuyaṣṭhī, Darbhamūla, Kamalanāla, Nilotpala mixed with honey and sugar-candy.[125]
2. Powder of Gavādanī (Indrāyaṇa) and Dāḍima should be prescribed with luke-warm water.[126]
3. Yavāgū (rice gruel) medicated with Mṛdvīkā and Kamala-nāla.[127]
4. Powder of Dāḍima, Jīraka, Nāgakeśar, etc. mixed with sugar and honey.[128]
5. Mayūrapicchabhasma with vyuṣita water.[129]
6. Water medicated with the bhasma of Vaṭa-kāṣṭha.[130]
7. Decoction of tender leaves of Āmra and Jumbū, Śālūka, Ativiṣā, Kṣīrī-vṛkṣa, Madhuyaṣṭhī, Kuśamūla, Cukra with sugar-candy and honey.[131]

These recipes have antiemetic property, thus help in preventing the vomiting. Some preparations like Yavāgū, etc.

may help in maintaining the electrolytic imbalance caused due to excessive vomiting.

Guda-Pāka

It may be considered as inflammatory condition of rectum including anal regions. The most common cause is change in pH of stool during diarrhoea, especially in newborns and infants or due to infection. Ancient scholars have noticed this complaint and prescribed its management.

Management

Suśruta opines that the treatment should be based on principle of treating vitiated pitta, the cause of guda-pāka.

Most of the texts have prescribed the following recipe for management of guda-pāka.

Solution of Rasāñjana should be prescribed for oral use, while its ointment should be applied locally. Paste prepared with Śankha, Madhuyaṣṭhī and Añjana.[132]

Utphullikā

Hārīta[133] has described utphullikā, not described by any previous scholars. He considers that consumption of vitiated breast milk by the child is the main cause of this troublesome disease.

It is characterised by ādhmāna, gases in the abdomen, difficulty in breathing, etc.

Treatment:

1. Raktamokṣaṇa should be performed by observing vitiation of doṣa.
2. Breast milk should be purified by prescribing decoction of Bilva-majjā, Pāṭhā, Sunṭhī, Marica, Pippalī, Kaṇṭakārīs (both) along with jaggery.

   This decoction is also useful in febrile condition.

3. The child should be exposed to fomentation (agni sweda) or abdomen should be cauterised like a dot.

F. DISORDERS OF RESPIRATORY SYSTEM

In children, most common symptoms of respiratory disorders are—Kāsa (cough) and Śvāsa (dyspnoea). Hiccā (Hiccup) has been described most of the time associated with Śvāsa. Ancient scholars have observed it very keenly, therefore, mentioned the specific treatments of Kāsa, Śvāsa and Hiccā, for chiidren.

Kāsa (Cough)

Kāsa is produced due to vitiation of Prāṇa vāyu along with Udāna vāyu. Caraka opines that vāyu impeded from below moves to the upper channels, attains character of Udāna vāyu and settles in throat and chest. Further it advances to all the orifices of head and filling them produces breaking pain and jerking in the whole body, particularly causing strain and shiftness in jaws, carotid region, orbits, eye balls, back, chest and sides. Thus dry and phlegmy cough arises. There is a peculiar type of sound during coughing which is very similar to the sound produced during hammering of broken bronze pot.[134]

Causes and Types of Kāsa

Caraka has mentioned the causes of kāsa according to vitiation of doṣa, while Suśruta has given only general causes.[135]

It is of 5 types—Vātika, paittika, kaphaja, kṣataja, and kṣayaja.

Features

Features of various types of kāsa roga are described in Table 31.

Table 31: Showing features of various types of kāsa

Type	*Parallel disease*	*Features*
1. Vātika	Acute bronchitis	Dry cough associated with headache, etc. pain in chest region. Attacks are very frequent, change in voice.
2. Paittika	Various inflammatory conditions of resp. tract	Burning sensation in chest, fever, dryness of mouth, feeling of thirst, yellow coloured vomits, anemia.
3. Kaphaja	Chronic bronchitis	Productive cough with thick sputum, headache, feeling of heaviness, etc.
4. Kṣataja	Due to injury of chest wall	Initially dry cough followed by haemoptysis, severe pain in chest, tenderness, attacks of pain, wheezing.
5. Kṣayaja	Due to various debilitating disease (e.g. Koch's, etc.)	Productive cough with thick and blood mixed sputum, associated with pain, burning and fever. Gradual wasting of body.

Now-a-days the cough has been considered as an unusual symptom in the new born. Cough with choaking, in a newborn infant may be due to tracheo-oesophageal fistula or oesophageal atresia, congenital laryngeal cleft or perforation of the pharynx. After the newborn period, the principal cause of cough is a respiratory infection, which include colds, pharyngitis, tonsillitis, laryngitis, tracheobronchitis, bronchiolitis, pneumonia, measles and whooping cough. Chronic cough may be due to a habit attention-seeking device. Other causes may include post nasal discharge, adenoids, asthma, bronchiolitis, pulmonary tuberculosis and congenital heart diseases.

Treatment

The recipes useful especially for children are as follows:

1. In śuṣka-kāsa (dry cough) the milk of dhātrī should be purified by prescribing her fried Pippalī (in ghṛta) with soup of Māṣa.[136]
2. Powder of Ativiṣā, Karkaṭaṣrangī and Pippalī or Mustā or powder of only Ativiṣā with honey may cure cough with fever and vomiting.[137]
3. Powder of Puṣkara-mūla, Ativiṣā, Karkaṭaṣrangī, Pippalī, Dhanvayāsa with honey, cures all types of cough.[138]
4. Powder of Drākṣā, Pippalī and Śuṇṭhī with honey.[139]
5. Puṣpa-keśara of Vyāghrī with honey.[140]
6. Powder of Haridrā, Pippalī, Kṛṣṇāñjana, Lājā, Karkasṭaśrangī and Marica with honey[141].
7. Powder of Harītakī, Vacā, Śuṇṭhī, Nāgaramothā and Karkaṭaṣrangī with equal quantity of jaggery.[142]

Śvāsa Roga (Dyspnoea)

The main feature of this disorder is difficulty in breathing (dyspnoea). Vitiated kapha blocks prāṇa-vaha srotasas producing śvāsa roga.

Āyurvedic scholars have described its five types.[143]

Classification is done on the basis of respiratory efforts. These are—Mahā śvāsa, Ūrdhva śvāsa, Chinna śvāsa, Tamaka and Kṣudra śvāsa.

Pratamaka and Santamaka śvāsa are complicated stage of Tamaka śvāsa.

In paediatric age group, the causes of dyspnoea may be grouped as follows:

(a) In newborns—respiratory distress syndrome, group A streptococcal infection, massive aspiration of amniotic fluid or meconium, transient tachypnoea.

(b) After newborn period—Acute dyspnoea may be due to the following causes:

  (i) Foreign body causing acute stridore.

  (ii) Pulmonary—pneumonia, asthma, asthmatic bronchitis, pneumothorax, massive collapse of lungs, pleural effusion, haemorrhage.

  (iii) Cardio-vascular-heart failure, paroxysmal tachycardia, congenital heart disease.

Chronic dyspnoea may be due to asthma, cystic fibrosis, emphysema, pleural effusion, corpulmonale, diaphragmatic hernia, severe chest deformity, RHD, myocarditis, anemia, obesity, ascites, renal failure, drugs, etc.

Features of śvāsa roga

Śvāsa roga have different features according to the type, which are summarised in the following Table 32.

Hiccā (Hiccough)

It is usually described along with śvāsa roga because their etiological factors are the same.

Vitiated Prāṇa vāyu and Udāna vāyu when gets activated together, obstructs, prāṇa, udāna and annavaha srotasa producing a typical sound.

Table 32 : Showing features of various types of śvāsa roga

Types	*Parallel condition*	*Features*
1. Mahāśvāsa	Biot's breathing	The patient becomes unconscious with open mouth and eyes, retention of urine and stool, loss of senses, difficulty in talking. The respiration can be watched from distance.
2. Ūdhva śvāsa	Stretorous breathing	In this condition expiration śvāsa is prolonged while inspiration is short, patient faint very often, restlessness, face appears white.
3. Chinna śvāsa	Cheyne stocks	Irregular respiratory efforts, difficulty in breathing may be due to pain in vital parts, delirium, restlessness, etc.
4. Tamaka śvāsa	Asthma	It mostly precipitate with pratiśyāya (coryza), feels uneasy during cough and may get relief after removing of sputum. Respiration is difficult during lying down posture while with some relief in sitting, presence of wheezing.
5. Kṣudra śvāsa	(exhertinal dyspnoea due to weakness)	Very mild type of dyspnoea usually associated with exercise.

It is of 5 types—Annaja, Mahatī, Gambhīrā, Yamalā and Kṣudrāśvāsa[144]

Young babies have frequently hiccough after a feed. Other causes include a subphrenic abscess, diaphragmatic pleurisy, cerebral tumor, peritonitis and ureamia.

Management of Śvāsa, Hiccā and Other Associated Respiratory Disorders

In ancient texts, the treatment of śvāsa roga is mentioned along with the treatment of kāsa and hiccā.

The following recipes are effective in both the conditions - śvāsa roga and hiccā:

1. Decoction of fruits, root and stem bark of Vṛhatī, Pippalī, Pippalāmūla, Tavakṣīra (Vaṃśalocana) with honey is effective in kāsa-śvāsa along with vaman, mūrcchā and fever.[145]
2. Powder of Citraka-mūla, Śuṇṭhī, Dantī-mūla and Indrāyaṇa with lukewarm water.[146]
3. Powder of Drākṣā, Yvāsa, Harītakī and Pippalī with ghṛta and honey or with honey alone, for 3-5 days.[148]
4. Powder of Dhānya and sugar with rice-water.[149]

G. DISEASES OF EYE

Care of eyes has been given much importance even in ancient period. Vāgbhaṭa has very rightly mentioned that one becomes useless without eyes. Various eye disorders and their management have been mentioned in Āyurvedic classics. According to Suśruta these are 76 in number, while 94 according to Vāgbhaṭa.

In children most common eye disorders have been described—Kukūṇaka, while others are—Pothakī, Pillikā, Upalepa, Kotha, etc.

General Principles of Treatment (Mentioned Especially by Kaśyapa):[150]

Kaśyapa has described general principles for treatment of various eye disorders affecting the children:

1. Dhātrī milk should be purified by performing śodhana therapy.
2. The drugs used for treating eye disorders should be mild, pure and in appropriate quantity. Strong medicines should be avoided, as far as possible.
3. Āścyotana—It is a special process used for instillation of medicine into eyes. In children it should be performed after 6 days of subsiding the features of acute stage, i.e., rāga (congestion), śotha (inflammation), śūla (pain) and aṣru srāva (lacrimation).

Following recipes may be used for this purpose:

(i) Dāru Haridrā, heated in sun light used with milk after rubbing it on the platform of copper and mixing with pond's water.

(ii) Water medicated with Harītakī, Āmalakī, Dāru-Haridrā and Madhuyaṣṭhī.

4. Saṃśamana therapy—Saṃaśamana therapy should be used, when the child is having dūṣikā, upalepa, draṣṭi-vyākulatā, arati, vartmaśotha, śiro-roga and when there is excessive secretion from eyes. It should be performed after passing of acute stage.

5. Dhātrī and child both should be prescribed congenial diet.
6. Use of Drugs:
   (a) Kaśyapa has mentioned use of six drugs for management of different eye disorders. These are—Cākṣuṣya, Puṣpaka, Mātā (Haritaki), Rocanā, Rasāñjana and Kaṭaka.

These should be used as a instillation, after rubbing in breast milk, in children upto the age of 6 months.

(i) Milk, honey, śanka nābhi and swarṇa-bhasma are dissolved in bronze pot and applied in eyes.

(ii) Paste of Cākṣuṣya prepared with special procedure, cures various complaints of eye, when used alone or in combination of other five drugs.

(iii) Powder of Puṣpaka should be applied in the afternoon or in night.

(iv) Combination of any two or three above drugs used as a paste prepared in milk and honey is more effective.

(b) Use of Pañcabhautika oil—Its use as nasal drops (nasya) is effective in most of the eye disorders. Apart from this it also acts as tonic for renovating intellect and strength.

7. Use of other preparations:

(i) Pillikā and Upalepa may be relieved by applying añjana, made of bark of Haridrā, Pippalī with superanatent of good quality of wine (Prasannā). Then eyes should be irrigated with sauvīraka.

(ii) For treatment of Timira and kotha roga—Use of tablets made by Pippalī, Ārdraka, Marica, Añjana,

Triphalā, Sankhanābhi, Saindhava, Tāmracūrṇa when used with water, cures timira while taken with juice of makoya, it is effective in kotha roga.

(iii) Excessive itching and timira—Oral use of latex of Karañja with ghṛta-manda and breast milk is very effective.

(iv) Severe pain in eyes—Use of Añjana prepared with Pippalī, Ārdraka, Tulasī, Kālītulasī and Kutheraka (a type of tulasī) with sura-maṇḍa.

(v) Irrigation (Pariṣeka) by lukewarm water medicated with Puṇḍarīka, Lodhra, Harīdrā, sugar and honey is effective in all eye disorders of children.

Kaśyapa has prescribed to use all the pariṣekas (irrigation) described in the treatment of eye complications during dentition.

(vi) An another Añjana made of Pippalī and Ārdraka is also effective in Pillikā.

(vii) Use of Guṭikās (tablets):

Kaśyapa has advised the use of tablets for management of general eye disorders of children. These are—Kokilā guṭikā, Lohitikā guṭikā.

(viii) Application of lepas (paste/ointment):

Kaśyapa and others have advised various lepas effective in treating various eye disorders:

(a) Paste made by ghṛta (one part) and honey (two parts) cures the problem very shortly.

(b) Lepa prepared with pasted Daśamūla, Nāgarmothā and Svarṇagairika in milk.[151]

(c) Pain in eye subsides by applying joint of Rasāñjana, pure Manahśilā, Sankhanābhi, Piccila taṇḍula and honey.[152]

(ix) Use of Añjanas:

(a) Pieces of copper are pasted with Marica, Ārdraka, curd and Kāñji for 7 consecutive days then these are grinded with curd and wicks are made for local application.

(b) Manahśilā, Śankhanābhi, Pippalī, Rasāñjana with honey.[153]

(c) Lodhra, Rasāñjana, Āmalakī and Svarṇagairika with honey.[154]

(x) Rasakriyās:

Kaśyapa has described two rasakriyās for relief of eye disorders:

(a) Triphalā, Añjana and Rasāñjana with honey.

(b) Pippalī, Ārdraka, Haritāla, Rasāñjana, buds of jasmine and jaggery with honey. It is known as kalyāṇikā-rasakriyā.

(xi) Other measures:

Kaśyapa has mentioned few other measures, which give relief in eye disorders:

(a) A fish named Mṛdagila is kept over eye, neck, etc. regions of body to get relief in eye disorders.

(b) A symbol of Kaṇṭaka (thorn) made by the paste of Alaka-taka and fresh roots of Vāstuka and Yava on the forehead of the child, suffering from eye disorders; was supposed to provide relief from symptoms.

Kukūṇaka

It is the commonest eye disorder of paediatric age group and especially of infancy. Its detailed description is available in Kaśyapa Saṃhitā, reference are also available in some other texts.

Etio-pathogenesis

There are two schools of thought regarding the concepts of etiological factors. Suśruta, Kaśyapa and Mādhava have considered it as a disorder of vitiated milk,[155] it is considered as a complication of dentition, by Vāgbhaṭa.[156] Suśruta has further described that it occurs due to vitiation of vāta, pitta, kapha and rakta doṣas.[157]

Kaśyapa has listed the factors, responsible for vitiation of breast milk and ultimately for development of Kukūṇaka.[158]

1. *Diet*

   (i) Consumption of too much sweet articles.

   (ii) Leafy vegetables.

   (iii) Milk and milk products, like butter, curd, etc.

   (iv) Products of flour.

   (v) Grinded tila.

   (vi) Sour articles like kāñjī.

2. *Mode of life*

   (i) Sleeping in day, after taking meal.

   (ii) Sudden arousal from bed on awakening.

Doṣas get vitiated, following above causes and spread in whole of the body, thus blocking milk-carrying channels. On consuming such vitiated milk for long time, the vitiated doṣa enters the body of child, producing this eye disorder by vitiating kapha and rakta.

Clinical Features

The child suffering with Kukūnaka may have following features:[159]

1. Excessive itching of eyes.
2. The child rubs eye balls, nose and forehead area.
3. Photophobia.
4. Excessive lacrimation.
5. Swelling of eye-lids.
6. Pain and heavyness in eye-lids.

All these above features are of Netra-abhiṣyanda described in Āyurvedic texts. With the modern point of view, Kukūṇaka may be considered as conjunctivitis, very common problem of childhood. The conjunctiva reacts to a wide range of bacterial and viral agents, allergens, irritants, toxins and systemic diseases.

Conjunctivitis in children may be of following types:

1. Acute purulent conjunctivitis
2. Opthalmia neonatorum
3. Epidemic keratoconjuncitivitis
4. Membranous or pseudomembranous conjunctivitis
5. Viral conjunctivitis
6. Allergic conjuncitivitis
7. Veneral conjunctivitis, and
8. Chemical conjunctivitis.

The following table provides the clues that which type of conjunctivitis is more closer to Kukūṇaka.

Table 33: Differential diagnosis of ocular-inflammation in children

Clinical features	*Kukūṇaka*	*Acute conju-nctivitis/ ophthalmia neonatorum*	*Acute Keratitis*	*Acute ureitis*
1. Discharge from eyes (Water/purulent)	+	+	+	+
2. Pain/foreign body sensation	+	+	+	+
3. Photophobia	+	±	+	+
4. Conjunctival redness	+	+	±	±

The above comparative study clarifies that the Kukūṇaka may not be equated with any one from the above mentioned conditions, while it will be more justifiable to say that Kukūṇaka is an acute ocular inflammatory condition, having generalised features of various varieties of conjunctivitis.

MANAGEMENT

Kaśyapa has very extensively described about the treatment of Kukūṇaka.[160] Other scholars have included various recipes in their description, for management of this problem.

Measures to be applied on Dhātrī

1. Dhātrī of affected child should be given emetics. After performing emesis and purgation properly, her breast

milk should be expressed out and she should be advised to take congenial diet.[161]

2. For dhātrī, Vāgbhaṭa[162] advised to offer ghṛta medicated with Khadira, Triphalā and Nimbapatra for snehana; Sarṣapa and rock salt for vamana; and decoction of Harītakī, Pippalī, Drākṣā for virecana.
3. Paste of Pippalī, Nāgaramothā, Haridrā and Daruharidrā should be pasted on breasts of dhātrī. Breasts should also be fumigated with ghṛta and Sarṣapa for purification of breast milk.
4. Dhātrī should remain clean. It may provide further spreading of the disease to the other children.

Measures applicable to the Child

1. Eyes of the child should be washed with water very thoroughly, after expressing out impure blood from the lids. This process may help in relieving the congestion.
2. After performing above procedures, drugs are applied in the eyes through Pariṣeka (irrigation), Aścyotana (instillation), application of lepas and Vartis (ointments).

(a) Pariṣeka (irrigation of eyes)

(i) Decoction of Eraṇḍa, Rohiṣa, Tvakṣīrī and Varuṇa.

(ii) Luke warm water prepared with Pauṇḍarīka, Lodhra, Haridrā, sugar and honey.

(iii) Luke warm water medicated with leaves of Āṭarūṣaka, Pauṇḍarīka and Nīlotpala, Madhuyaṣṭhī and rock salt.

(iv) Water medicated with decoction of Guḍūcī and solution of Kuṣṭha and jaggery .

(v) Eyes should be irrigated with luke warm decoction of Dvīpī (Citraka) and Śatru (Amlavetasa).

(b) Aścyotana (Instillation)

Following preparations are useful as instillation:

(i) The juice extracted from Phaṇijjhaka (a type of Tulasī) and Tulasī should be used after mixing it with jati (juice of Jasmine leaves), Prasannā (a type of wine), Maṇḍa and Madhuyaṣṭhī.

(ii) Juice of Bharangarāja and Bilva, after mixing with Surāmaṇḍa.

(iii) Goat's milk medicated with grinded Kapittha, Bilva, and Khadira or with Kapitha, Ajājī and leaves of Tulasī.

(iv) Goat's milk medicated with Madhuyaṣṭhī and Dāruharidrā.

(v) Application of Rasāñjana (procured from hills of Tārkṣya) and mixed with honey.

(vi) Sugar, Ārdraka, Gopitta (Gorocana) and Rasāñjana with honey.

(vii) Grinded Haridrā and Sankhanābhi mixed with little amount of milk.

(viii) Instillation prepared with Puṭapāka with Śuṇṭhī, Bhrangarāja, Haridrā and rock-salt.

(c) Añjana

(i) Añjana prepared with Haridrā, Dāruharidrā, Lodhra, Madhuyaṣṭhī, Kuṭakī, Nimba (Kaṭu) and Tāmra-bhasma.

(ii) Skin of Bṛhatī and Añjana in equal parts, is very effective in Kukūṇaka.

(iii) Añjana prepared by grinded Viḍanga, Hartāla, Manhśilā, Dāruharidā, and Svarṇa-gairika in Kāñjī.

(iv) Añjana prepared with powder of Sudarśana-mūla.

(d) Lepa

(i) Application of paste prepared with Bhrangarāja, Nīla, Tulasī, Śweta Sarṣapa and Haridrā.

(ii) Paste prepared by adding grinded Padmākha, Utpala, Madhuyaṣṭhī and sugar in goat's milk.

(iii) Paste of Ārdraka, Mañjiṣṭhā, Kārpāsa and Kulaka (Paṭola).

(iv) Use of lepa prepared with Harītakī, Vibhītakī, Āmalakī, Lodhra, Punarnavā, Śuṇṭhī, Brahtīs (both) in equal quantity with water.

(v) Lepa of ghṛta and elephant's urine.

(e) Use of Vartis

For application in eyes, Vartis should be rubbed with water on a stone. The ointment prepared is used for application. Kaśyapa has prescribed to use Añjana-varti for the treatment of Kukūṇaka.[162]

H. SKIN DISORDERS

Indian knowledge about health and ill-health of the skin goes as far back as the Vedic period. In Ṛg Veda terms 'Casma' and 'tvacā' have been found to denote the skin. Various diseases of skin like Kuṣṭha, Kilāsa, Palita have also been described. Atharva Veda has added some more new diseases, like Pania, Aruṣa, Vidradha, Apacī, etc. However, description of skin disorder, manifesting especially to the children have not been described in Vedas but discussed in Āyurvedic texts.

The children are of delicate nature, therefore, easily affected from various diseases, especially of skin because it comes in direct contact of external environment. Skin of child is also not fullly mature and have following differences from adults:

1. Children's skin is much thin, soft and sensitive.
2. There is no proper contact in epidermis and dermis.
3. Blood supply is not adequate.

4. Sweat glands are not fully matured.
5. Heat regulation capacity is also poor due to deficiency in subcutaneous fat.

Due to these above differences, there are some specific disorders of skin, which are more common in children and their references are available in ancient Indian literature. These are:

1. Ahipūtanā
2. Carmadala
3. Śakunī graha
4. Others—Visarpa, Pāmā, Vicarcikā, Mahāpadma, Pittadagdha skin, Vṛṇa, Piḍikā, etc.

In Āyurvedic texts a general term, 'Kuṣṭha' has been given for skin disorders.

Ahipūtanā

Infants are said more vulnerable to this disease. Vāgbhata has mentioned various synonyms for it, like Mātṛkā doṣa, Praṣṭhāru, Gudakanda and Anāmaka.[163]

Etiological Factors:

Suśruta and Vāgbhaṭa both have considered almost similar factors, responsible for development of this disorder. The most important cause is improper cleaning of napkin area (gudā), which remains wet with stool and sweat. Other cause may be consumption of vitiated breast milk by the child.[164]

Clinical Features[165]

It is a rakta and kapha disorder, therefore have the features accordingly.

1. Itching in the napkin area.

2. Formation of sphoṭa (papule/pustule) and there may be oozing, due to excessive scratching.
3. Ulcers may be formed, which may have various complications.

This disease may be considered as 'Napkin rash,' especially affecting the napkin area of the infants. The main cause is wetting of this area with urine. Local symptoms develop in the skin, due to effect of ammonia, formed by the fermentation of the urea, present in urine. Initially, the skin is inflammed with itching which further develop papules/pustules and ultimately ulcers. There may be secondary infection of candida albicans.

Table 34: Showing comparison of Ahipūtanā with Napkin Rashes

Etiological factors & Clinical features	*Ahipūtanā*	*Napkin rash*
Age—Childhood	+	+
Etiological factors:		
Improper cleaning of napkin area	+	+
Affected area—Napkin area	+	+
Clinical features:		
Inflammation	+	+
Itching	+	+
Sphoṭa (Papule/pustule)	+	+
Ulcers	+	+

Treatment:

The treatment of Ahipūtanā includes purification of vitiated breast milk, local application of medicine on affected part along with drugs/recipes for oral use of the child.

1. *Purification of vitiated milk:*

Suśruta and Vāgbhaṭa both are of opinion that the vitiated milk of dhātrī should be purified whose child is suffering from Ahipūtanā, for this purpose drugs should be prescribed which are Pitta-Kapha Śāmaka.[166]

2. *Local Treatment:*

(a) Irrigation/cleaning—The affected part should be washed or irrigated with water medicated with decoction of Triphalā, Badara and Plakṣa.[167]

(b) Local application of Lepa (Ointments):

(i) Kāsīsa, Gorocana, Tuttha, Haritāla and Rasāñjana or bark of Badara or rock salt grinded in Kāñjī.[168]

Some texts have used Manahiśilā for Haritāla.[169]

(ii) Use of Rasāñjana with honey.[170]

(iii) Lepa of Asana (Vijaya sāra).[171]

(iv) Sankha-bhasma, Sauvīrāñjana and Madhuyaṣṭhī.[172]

(c) Dusting: Suśruta has advised that dusting of medicated powder should be done, when the ulcers are under process of healing.

(i) Finely powdered Kapāla (red hotted earthen pot) and Tuttha.[173]

(ii) Powder of Kāsīsa, Gorocana, Tuttha, Manahśilā, Haritāla and Rasāñjana.

(iii) Powdered Sārivā and Sankha-nābhi.[174]

(d) Blood letting by application of leech.[175]

Vāgbhaṭa has advised for blood-letting by application of leech, if there is excessive inflammation and itching.

3. *Oral Administrations:*

(i) Ghṛta medicated with Paṭola-patra, Triphalā and Rasāñjana.[176]

(ii) Water prepared with Śveta Candana should be advised for oral administration.[177]

Carmadala

It is one of the peculiar disease of childhood, affecting mostly infants (kṣīrāda and kṣīrānnāda). Kaśyapa[178] has described it in very detail, however, Caraka and Suśruta have just mentioned its name alongwith very few characteristic features and included in the list of Kṣudra Kuṣṭha.[179]

It may be considered as infantile atopic dermatitis.

Definition:

Kaśyapa has defined it as '*Carmadalamiti Carmāvaḍarḍāta.*' Cracking of skin is the main feature of this disease. It has predominance of Vāta.[180]

Etiopathogenesis:

Carmadala affects only to the children, who are Kṣīrapa or Kṣīrānnāda, due to consumption of vitiated milk. It's incidences are very less in children, whose main diet is cereals (annāda).

Because the skin, bones and dhātus of these (annāda) children are more stable and physically strong due to performing vrious exercises. Due to unstable dhātus, children (Kṣīrāda and Kṣīrānnāda) are deficient in bala (immunity), therefore, more susceptible for this disease.[181]

Other factors described in the etiology of this disease are:[182]

1. Unstability of dhātus.
2. Putting on cloths and keeping in lap for a long time.
3. Due to effect of exposure to hot air, strong sunlight, application of poultice and due to improper hygiene (not cleaning his urine and stool properly).
4. Excessive sweating.

5. Applying much pressure by hands on the child, and application of anointment.
6. Hereditary (Kulaja).

It may be very well explained that why this disease is more common in Kṣīrāda and Kṣīrānnāda. Among these some children are more sensitive to the milk protein. On consuming milk these children may develop various features including of skin. Annāda and adults have no incidence, because most of the children after attaining the age of 2 years develop sātmyatā (acceptability) for various milk proteins and food allergens. This may be the cause for not involving the older children from this disease.

Infantile atopic dermatitis, parallel to Carmadala, has been also considered hereditary. In a study it has been demonstrated that in 70% cases, there was positive family history for this disease (Rajka G. 1960).

Clinical Features

Caraka[183] is of opinion that the skin lesions (sphoṭa) are reddish, painful and having itching; while Suśruta[184] has described that there is excessive burning, pain and itching in palms and soles. There is feeling of dryness (Coṣa). According to Kaśyapa[185] it affects the face, neck, hands, foot, groin region, back and joints (folds of skin).

Parallel disease infantile dermatitis also starts from face. Initially the affected skin is inflammed then small boils appear which later on burst and there is crest formation. Pain and itching are associated features. In later stage, it spreads in other body parts like forehead, neck, wrist and arm, leg and sometimes in groin region. In chronic stage, the skin becomes dry and eczematization occurs. These features simultaneously subsides after the age of 2 years.

Table 35: Showing comparison of Carmadala with Infantile atopic dermatitis

Etiological factors & Clinical features	*Diseases*	
	Carmadala	*Infantile atopic dermatitis*
Age		
Kṣīrapa or Kṣīrānnāda	+	+
Causative factors:		
1. Milk and food disorders (allergy)	+	+
2. Excessive wearing of cloths, anointment	+	+
3. Hereditary	+	+
Clinical features:		
1. Inflammation	+	+
2. Boils, itching and pain	+	+
3. Cracking of skin	+	+

The above table clearly indicates the close resemblance of Carmadala with Infantile atopic dermatitis.

Types

Kaśyapa has described its four types—Vātika, Paittika, Śleṣmika and Sannipātika.[186]

Various etiological factors along with clinical features of above four types of Carmadala are described in Table 36.

Table 36: Etiological factors and clinical features of various types of Carmadala.[187]

Type	*Etiological factors (in dhātrī)*	*Clinical features (in child)*
1. Vātika	Rūkṣa āhāra-vihāra, anointment, fast, too much walking and exercise by mother	Hard bluish spots with boils, oozing of foamy liquid, tingling sensation, loose stools of various colours, Kampana, Mukha Śoṣa and Romaharṣa.
2. Paittka	Uṣṇa, amla, lavaṇa, kaṭu and vidāhi diet, Adhya-śana, anger, etc.	The spots may be reddish, bluish, yellowish with foul smelling. Affect skin and burn. Loose stools grey or yellow coloured, Gudapāka, Dāha, Mukha śoṣa, vomiting, yellowish face.
3. Śleṣmika	Use of articles which are guru, amla, lavaṇa, madhura, abhiṣyandi and excessive sleeping in day	The spots are white coloured, equal to sarṣapa, less in quantity and less pain and burning. Loose stools whitish, vomiting, etc.
4. Sanni-pātika	All the factors respon-sible for vitiating all the three doṣas	Spots are of various colours, very foul smelling secretions, dyspnoea, excessive weeping, refusal to suck breast. Loose stools - reddish or bluish.

These above types may be considered as different stages of this diseases (infantile atopic dermatitis).

Conditions making the disease complicated: Carmadala becomes more complicated and difficult to treat, if it is associated with vomiting, thirst, fever, distension, oedema, hiccough, dyspnoea, etc.[188]

These above conditions appear due to secondary bacterial infection in the skin lesion. The associated secondary GIT infection may cause loose stools, vomiting and ultimately dehydration. Naturally, the treatment will be more complicated due to these.

Principles of Treatment

Kaśyapa opines that this disease should be treated very carefully because there are more chances of recurrence.[189]

Since no specific treatment has been described for the affected child, except purification of breast milk of his dhātrī. It indicates that disease is self-limiting, therefore, its treatment is not required. Purification of milk is done only to prevent its further extension because there are more chances of recurrence as described by Kaśyapa.

For purifying the breast milk dhātrī (mother) should be given śodhan therapy, according to vitiation of doṣa. Dhātrī should be induced for vamana and virecana after performing snehana for pitta vitiated carmadala. For elimination of doṣas, vomiting is induced by administering a mixture of decoction of Nimba and paste of Pippalī or decoction of Pippalī with lavaṇa. Purgation may be induced by offering her decoction made of Drākṣā, juice of sugar-cane and Harītakī or Drākṣā and Āmalakī or pulp of fruits of Amalatāsa and milk, followed by saṃsarjana.

For elimination of vāta doṣa, snehana and swedana are performed followed by administration of ghṛta medicated with Nīlikā or Trivṛtta. Various lepa, periṣeka and abhyanga are advised to treat vātika carmadala.

In kaphaja carmadala, vitiated kapha is eliminated by inducing emesis on administering solution of Pippalī in lukewarm water, followed by Śirovirecana.[190]

Visarpa

It has been described by most of the scholars that Visarpa affects mostly to elder persons, but in opinon of Kaśyapa, small children are more prone to this disorder[191]. Therefore, he has described it in detail especially in relation to children.

Definition

Caraka[192] has justified the name of this disease as 'Visarpa' because of its nature of spreading rapidly. Suśruta and Kaśyapa are of similar opinion.[193]

Caraka has mentioned that rakta (blood), lasikā (lymph glands), tvacā (skin) and māṃsa (muscles) are dūṣya; while vāta, pitta and kapha are doṣa, responsible for causing this disease.[194]

Etiopathogenesis

In the opinion of Caraka, regular consumption of articles which are lavaṇa, amla, kaṭu, ūṣṇa and tīkṣṇa, may cause this disease.[195] Kaśyapa has given a list of etiological factors.[196]

1. Injury—Various injuries causing fracture, laceration and cutting of the part.
2. Diet.
   (i) Consumption of sour articles, like-kāñjī, sauvīra, etc.
   (ii) Use of Tila, Kulattha, flesh of animals and bird living in marshy land (ānūpa pradeśa) and in water (audaka), onion, garlic and other articles which are guru, abhiṣyandi and paryuṣita.
   (iii) Consumption of vitiated breast milk.
   (iv) Polluted air, water, toxic food substances, etc.

The bacterias (Haemolytic streptococcus) may invade through broken skin (by any trauma). Since small children have low resistance power (Ksīṇa bala), thus in these, the invasive properties of H. Streptococcus are high, resulting a rapidly spreading disease—Erysipelas, which may be considered equivalent to Visarpa.

Types of Visarpa and their Features:

Caraka, Kaśyapa and Vāgbhaṭa[197] (7 types)	*Suśruta*[198] (5 types)
1. Vātika	1. Vātaja
2. Paittika	2. Pittaja
3. Kaphaja	3. Kaphaja
4. Vāta-pittaja (āgneya)	4. Sannipātaja
5. Sannipātaja	5. Kṣataja
6. Kapha-vātaja (granthi)	
7. Pitta-kaphaja (Kardamaka)	

1. Vātika Visarpa—The associated symptoms are pain, inflammation, pain like piercing needles, fatigue and roma-harṣa, etc.
2. Pittaja Visarpa—It spreads very rapidly and there are features like Pittaja-jvara, eruption (red colour).
3. Kaphaja Visarpa—Itching, smoothness and other features of Kaphaja-jvara.
4. Sannipāta Visarpa—This type of visarpa have combined features of all above three types.
5. Vāta-pittaja (Āgneya)—The affected part become blackish, bluish or reddish and rapid appearance of blisters. It spreads very rapidly in vital parts (marmas). Other associated symptoms are fever, vomiting,

diarrhoea, thirst, giddiness, weak digestive power (agnimanda) and anorexia, etc.

6. Kapha-vātaja (Granthi) Visarpa—The main feature is chain of granthis (multiple laymphadenitis).
7. Pitta-kaphaja (Kardama) Visarpa—Boils appear yellowish, reddish or brownish and very foul smelling. The associated features are—fever, dulness, headache, weakness, anorexia, hallucination, syncope, etc.
8. Kṣataja Visarpa—This type has been added by Suśruta. It spreads following an injury and have boils, like kulatha. There is burning, inflammation and fever.

Principles of Management

Kaśyapa has given following general principles for management of visarpa:[199]

1. The treatment should be initiated in an early stage when doṣas are slightly aggravated and are in the outer part of the body, not deep seated.
2. Initially treatment should be started as Vamana and Virecana to the dhātrī for purifying the vitiated doṣas and to purify the breast milk.
3. Considering time, Langhana (fasting) should be advised, which should be followed by drinking of decoction.
4. Further the patient should be treated by Pradeha, Pariṣecana, Sneha, Abhyanga and Rektamokṣaṇa.
5. Use of purāṇa sarpi (old ghṛta) or Kumbha sarpi is very effective in vātika-visarpa. Other types of visarpas should be treated according to vitiation of doṣa. Kaśyapa has given its detailed description.
6. Use of congenial diet and mode of life—Old Yavānna, Śāli rice, Mudga, Masūra, Hareṇu, meat of birds and animals (living in forests).

Caraka has contraindicated the use of Vidāhī diet, sleeping in day, anger, exercise, exposure to sun and agni.[200]

Mahāpadma

Vāgbhaṭa has added a specific type of Visarpa, known as Mahāpadma. It occurs due to vitiation of all the three doṣas and affect especially sira and vasti pradesa. The skin becomes red, like—Padma (Kamala), therefore, termed as Mahāpadma. Some times it involves other body parts also. It has been considered very difficult to treat.[201]

Treatment

Vāgbhaṭa has mentioned no any specific treatment, however, Vangasena has prescribed few preparation which are used as local application and some for oral administration.[202]

(a) *Local Application*

(i) Paste of Sārivā, Utpala, Kalhar, Bhadraṣrī, Mustā, Candana, Prapauṇḍarīka, Mañjiṣṭhā, Madhuyaṣṭhī and Sarṣapa.

(ii) Application of Mahāpadma ghṛta, as massage.

(iii) Paste of Nygrodha, Udumbara, Aśvattha, Plakṣa, Vetasa, bark of Jambū, Madhuyaṣṭhī, Mañjiṣṭhā, Candana, Khasa and Padmākha.

It relieves inflammation, burning and helps in healing of ulcers.

(b) *Oral recipes*

Decoction of Paṭola-patra, Triphalā, bark of Nimba and Haridrā.

Paścādruja (Vṛṇa Paścādruja)

It is a disorder appeared due to consumption of vitiated breast milk and described by Vangasena.[203]

Clinical Features

The vitiated pitta produces following features in the child.

1. The anal region become reddish (similar to abdomen of leech who has recently sucked the blood) with burning pain.
2. Formation of ulcers.
3. Colour of stool become yellowish and there may be constipation.
4. It may be associated with fever and cough.

It is very troublesome disorder.

Treatment

1. Blood letting should be done by application of leech. It may relieve congestion, thus reducing inflammation and burning.
2. Cleaning of anal region with lukewarm decoction of Pañcakṣīrī vṛkṣa.
3. Local application of paste of Madhuyaṣṭhī.
4. Paste of Candana, both Sārivā and Sankha-nābhi should be used as local application or may be used as avaleha.
5. Tablets (Guṭikās) made by fine powdered flowers of Asana (Vijaya Sāra) taken with rice water may relieve from the trouble.

Śakunī Graha

It is an infective disorder. In Āyurvedic texts it has been described under graha rogas.[204] Involvement of skin is the chief complaint. It can be equated with Impetigo, described in modern texts.

It will be discussed in detail under the heading Bāla grahas.

Paridagdha Chavi

Appearance of burn mark due to Pitta, etc. factors, it is termed as Paridagdha Chavi, and mostly observed in children.

Vāgbhaṭa has prescribed to apply paste of Dūrvā, Tila, Utpala, leaves of Śamī, stem-bark of Śirīṣa, Ananta-mūla, Madhuyaṣṭhī and Khasa; on affected skin.[205]

Ajagallikā

Some children may develop small piḍikās equal to the size of Mudga. These are smooth, painless, skin coloured and said to occur with Kapha and Vāta. Suśruta has listed it in 'Kṣudra Rogas.'[206]

Treatment

Only local treatment has been prescribed.[207]

1. Application of ointment of Śukti, Svarjikā Kṣāra and Yavakṣāra.
2. Paste of Śyāmā, Lāngalī and Pāṭhā for local application.

Arakīlikā

The child when usually put the powder of bricks on his head, consumes the seed of Trapuṣa and Ervāruka, take diet which increases meda and sleep in day. By these factors, the vitiated meda with vāyu, come into skin; causes appearance of very small and few eruptions, which may later on become enlarged in size equivalent to Drākṣā.

Treatment

These should be cauterised by application of ūṣṇa-sneha or gada or kṣāra should be applied after excising them. Kṣāra-sūtras may also be used later on the processes described for management of vṛṇa are performed.

This disorder has been described by Kaśyapa.[208]

Āmaccheda

The children, which are more active and use to move very frequently here and there, they may harm themselves by various objects like wood, bricks and instruments, etc.; producing wounds.

Treatment

Kaśyapa has prescribed following treatment for āmaccheda.[209]

1. This should be cleaned by lukewarm water.
2. Bleeding may be checked by application of cold water.
3. Use of Svedana, Dahana and Kṣāra may be applied, if required. These processes may prevent the infections like tetanus, which is very prevalent with such type of injuries.

Dadru

Kaśyapa[210] has described that the child may suffer from dadru, due to following etiological factors:

1. In winter season, when the child usually sleeps in the lap, therefore, not provide time to change the wet cloths, very frequently.
2. Bearing too much cloths.
3. Sleeping on tṛṇa or grass.
4. The child is not given bath and anointment.

The above factors may help in infestation of worms, ticks and lices in the body; producing dadru. Scabies and fungal infections are more common with the above mentioned etiology.

Treatment

1. The affected child should be massaged and bathed daily.

2. Fumigation helps to kill the micro or macro-organisms, responsible for symptoms.
3. Bed and cloths should be changed daily.

Romāntikā

Mādhava has first time included this disease in his description.Its features are similar to the disease which is now-a-days known as measles.

Initially the child suffer from fever, cough and anorexia followed by appearance of very small, red coloured pidikās (rashes/macules) due to vitiation of kapha and pitta. This disease may be complicated with cough, hiccough, high fever, weakness, thirst, burning, excessive secretion from mouth, nostrils and eyes, difficulty in respiration with stridor.[211]

In measles prodromal features are high fever, coryza, conjunctivitis, photophobia, irritant cough. Koplic spots appear opposite to the lower molar and usually disappear within 18-20 hours. The rashes on body appears usually on the 4th or 5th day as faint macule on the lateral borders of the neck along the hairline and progressively involves the face, trunk and abdomen. When the rash appears in the lower extremities, it begins to clear on the face and disappears in the course of 3-6 days. The child look irritable, listless, red eyed with puffy eye lids, with copious thin nasal discharge.

The chief complications of measles are pneumonia, gastroenteritis, otitis media, and encephalitis.

Vṛṇa

Suśruta has defined vṛṇa as—one which smashes the body (*Vṛṇa-gātra vicūrṇane*) or which causes discolouration (*Vraṇāyatita vṛṇah*).[212]

Vṛṇa are of two types—Nija and Āgantuja.[213]

1. Nija Vṛṇa—These are doṣaja vṛṇa—i.e., vātika, paittika, kaphaja, dwidoṣaja and sannipātika.
2. Āgantuja Vṛṇa—Āgantuja Vṛṇa may be caused by bhagna (fracture), viddha, pātana, dagdha, chinna, nispiṣta and injury by śastra, tṛṇa, kāṣṭha, agni, viṣa, danta, nakha, śāpa, mantra, etc.

Kaśyapa has described features and management of various types of Vṛṇa, in children because there are much chances of injury in them.[214]

Table 37: Showing clinical features and management of various types of vṛṇa in children.

Type of Vṛṇa	*Clinical features*	*Management*
1. Vātika	Stambha (spasticity), Kaṭhinatā (hardness), alpasrāva (less secretions), śūla, toda (piercing pain), sphuraṇa (throbbing), kaṣāya (astringent taste)	Snehapāna, snigdha diet, snigdha upanāha snigdha sveda, ūṣṇa pariṣeka and use of madhura, amla and lavaṇa articles.
2. Paittika	Jvara (fever), dāha (burning), moha, tṛṣṇā (thirst), Āśu-pāka (easy suppuration), lālimā (inflammation), avadāraṇa (bursting of boil), feeling of anorexia and foul smelling	Pariṣeka by cold water and milk, śītala, lepa, use of madhura kaṣāya and tikta articles, use of ghṛta, mudga, śāli rice, meat-soup of Jāngala birds and animals
3. Kaphaja	Stimista (stickyness), Śītalatā (coldness), mṛdutā (softness), manda vedanā (mild pain), snigdhitā (smoothness), pāṇḍura (yellowish in colours), cirkāritta (chronic), srāvādhikya (secretion)	Use of ūṣṇa, tikta kaṭu, kaṣāya, kṣāra articles, saṃśodhans upanāha, svedana, Pariṣeka by uṣṇa jala, langhan (fast), sarāvaṇa and bandhana (bandage)
4. Dvidoṣaja and Sannipātika	These types have mixed type of features	Treatment according to predominance of doṣa.

General Principles of Treatment

For management of Vṛṇa, several processes have been described by various scholars. Caraka has given 36, Suśruta 60 processes (Upakrama) while Kaśyapa has described very few, applicable to the children and his mother. It includes Saṃśodhana (purification), Banadhan (bandage), Utklinna māmsa prakṣālana, Kalka-prāṇidhāna(application of paste), Śodhana, Ropaṇa and Savarṇīkaraṇa.

Srāvaṇa (drainage), Pātana (incision), Dāhana (cauterization), Sīvana (suturing), Eṣaṇa (probing) should be avoided in small children.

If wound is on vital part (marma), then it should be avoided for incision, etc. procedures. These should be slightly rubbed and bandaged with curd (cow's) and salt. However, other wounds may be incised by an expert surgeon, keeping in view the condition of child. Because a previously anemic child may become more serious by bleeding occurred due to improper incision.[215]

Piḍikās

Caraka and Suśruta, both have described that in an adult, piḍikās may appear, as a complication of prameha.[216] Kaśyapa has described 8 types of Piḍikās affecting the children. These are Śarāvikā, Kacchapikā, Jālinī, Sarsapikā, Alājī, Vidradhi, Vinitā and Arunṣikā.

Description of these piḍikās, their clinical features and treatment is summarised in Table 38.

Table 38: Features and treatment of 'Aṣṭa-piḍikās' (Described by Kaśyapa[217])

Doṣa vitiated	*Piḍikā*	*Features*	*Principles of treatment*
Kaphaja	1. Śarāvikā	Depressed in centre.	Initially snehana is done, followed by virecana. Then various processes should be performed. Unripened boils should be subsided by pariṣeka, pralepa, use of ghṛta and congenial diet.
	2. Kacchapikā	Smooth and elevated.	
	3. Jālinī	Full of veins & with multiple small seive like apertures.	
Pittaja	1. Sarṣapikā	Equal to size of sarṣapa, many in number and frequent suppuration.	
	2. Alajī	Suppurate, very easily spreads and have various complications,	
	3. Vidradhi	These appear mostly on joints and on vital parts (marmas), excessive burning, involvement of māmsa dhātu	
Vātaja	4. Vinitā	Most common site is abdomen and back, appear dark, bluish and much painful.	
Tridoṣaja	Arunṣikā (4 types according to further predominance of doṣas)	These mostly appears on head and may be considered as seborrhic dermatitis	(i) Shaving of scalp, cleaning and application of medicated oil. (ii) In painful conditions anointment

(a) Vātika	Śūla, toda, āṭopa, sphuraṇa, ānaha, parna.	of tila, or butter should be done.
(b) Paittika	Jvara, traṣṇā, dāha, moha, mada and pratapa	(iii) In case, these contain blood, then these should be removed by a sharp instrument and ointment made of cow's milk and cow's urine (in equal quantity), should be applied.
(c) Śleṣmika	Śīta, picchila, kleda, aruci and stimitata	
(d) Samdoṣaja	Symptoms may be of combined types.	

I. DISEASES AND SYMPTOMS RELATED TO URINARY SYSTEM

The most common urinary diseases or symptoms are prevalent in children even today, after passing of the period of thousands of years. The symptoms/disorders observed by ancient scholars are:

1. Mūtraśmarī (Vesical calculus)
2. Mūtrakṛccha (Dysuria)
3. Mūtragraha (Retention of urine)
4. Śaiyyāmūtratā (Bed wetting)

Mūtrāśmarī

Suśruta[218] is of opinion that children may also suffer from mūtrāśmarī (vesical calculus). He has described four types of aśmarīs—vātika, paittika, ślesmika and Sukraja. Among these, first three are said to occur in children, while the last, i.e., śukrāśmarī is not found in children because of non-formation of śukra in them.

The incidences of mūtrāśmarī is high in children because their body and urinary bladder is small and there is less deposition of māṃsa.

Etiological Factors:

Suśruta has described following etiological factors, responsible for formation of mūtrāśmarī.[219]

1. Not performing purification of body by vamana, virecana, etc. process of pañcakarma.
2. Consumption of non-congenial diet-excessive use of śīta (cold), snigdha(smooth), guru(heavy), madhura (sweet) diet.
3. Performing non-congenial activities and mode of life, i.e., sleeping in day, adhyaśana, etc.

Formation of Calculus:

Suśruta has described that śleṣmā acts as a base (āśraya) in formation of mūtrāśmarī (V. calculus). He has simplified the concept regarding formation of aśmarī, with an example, and explained that as the water filled in new pitcher precipitate some impurities when kept for long time. In the same way due to various precipitating factors (as described above), the aśmarī may be produced by urine, in the bladder.[220]

A primary vesical calculus is one that develops in sterile urine. It often originates in a kidney and passes down the ureter to the bladder, where it enlarges. The secondary vesical calculus occurs in the presence of infection. A vesical calculus can also occur by the deposition of urinary salts upon a foreign body in the bladder. This description very clearly proves the theory of Suśruta, mentioned for formation of vasical calculus.

Prodromal Features:

The affected child may have following prodromal features.[221]

1. Pain in vasti (pubic region), vasti śira, vastidvāra and in penis and testicles (referred pain).

2. Pain during micturation (dysuria) and it depends upon vitiation of doṣas.
3. Fever and weakness (due to exhaustion).
4. The colour of urine may be also changed according to vitiation of doṣas.

Clinical Features:

1. During micturation there may be pain in nābhi (umbilical area), vasti (pubic region) or mehana (penis).
2. Improper micturation due to obstruction.
3. Hematuria.
4. Abnormal current of urine, while voiding.
5. Urine—In appearance, the urine is clear but it may contain small gravels/particles of sikatā (sand).

Vāgbhaṭa has described similar features as described above by Suśruta, however, Kaśyapa in Vedanādhyāya has also given some general features of aśmarī. He has added one specific feature, that the child suffering from mutraśmarī, cries excessively. Other features are similar to Suśruta.[222]

Suśruta has mentioned specific features according to predominance of doṣa. These are summarised in the following Table 39.

Table 39: Types of mūtrāśmarī and their specific feature[223]

Type of Aśmarī	*Physical appearance*	*Specific features*	*Comments*
1. Vātāśmarī	Aśmarī is blackish, rough, irregular and may have various spikes	Very severe pain	It is formed by oxalate of lime
2. Pittāśmarī	Reddish, Yellowish or Blackish and similar to size of Bhallātaka seed.	Pain with burning	Uric acid calculus

3. Kaphaśmarī	Whitish, smooth and large size,	Pain like piercing by needless, feeling of heaviness and cold.	Phosphate calculus

Management:

Suśruta was very clear that the medical treatment may be effective only in acute condition, while in chronic cases surgery should be the choice.[224]

(a) *Medical management*—As soon as the prodromal features are noticed, various purificatory measures like snehana, svedana etc. along with medicines should be prescribed. The treatment given only in such early stage may be effective to cure it completely.[225]

(b) *Surgical management*—Various steps of surgical procedures and post-operative care have been described by Suśruta.[226] However, Kaśyapa[227] has contraindicated the forceful extraction of aśmarī, in small children, as it may cause mūtra-srāvī vṛṇa.

Mūtrakṛccha (Dysuria)

Mūtrakṛccha is a condition of painful micturation (dysuria). It is the main feature of aśmarī.[228] Various scholars have classified the problem, accordingt to vitiation of doṣas. Caraka has described its 8 types.[229] Similarly Suśruta and Kaśyapa have also mentioned its 8 types but with different names.[230]

Kaśyapa has mentioned the feature of different types of mutrakṛccha, affecting the children.[231]

Table 40: Features related to various types of mūtrakrccha (as described by Kaśyapa)

Type of Mūtrakṛccha	*Probable equivalent disease*	*Features*
1. Vātika	Urethral stricture	1. Urine appears foamy and comes in little amount 2. Pain during micturation 3. Constipation 4. Colour of urine—reddish and blackish
2. Paittika	Infection	1. Burning and painful micturation 2. Urine is hot with vapours 3. Sweating on face during micturation 4. Colour of urine—yellowish.
3. Kaphaja	Chyluria	1. Polyurea 2. Urine is concentrated (ghana) 3. Comparatively less difficulty during micturation 4. Heaviness and inflammation in Vasti pradeśa 5. Colour of urine—Whitish.

Dvandvaja and Sannipātaja have features according to predominance of doṣas. Similarly, Raktaja mūtrakṛccha have features similar to Pittaja mūtrakṛccha except colour, which is reddish due to blood.

These above features may be associated with Urinary Tract infections, Urinary Calculus, etc.

General Principles of Treatment

Kaśyapa has mentioned general principles for treatment of mūtrakṛccha.[232]

1. The child should be purified by using mild procedures (Vamana, Virecana, etc.).
2. The diet and drugs should be opposite as used in Kuṣṭha disease thus avoiding samgrāhī and vidāhī articles.
3. Congenial diet should contain sweet substances; various preparations of sugar-cane juice, trapuṣa, ghṛta and milk.

   Rice gruel (Yavāgū) medicated with Karañja, Nigarbhā, Kārpāsa, Śigru, Gokṣura, Mṛnāls, Utpala, rock salt, etc. should be given to child.
4. Decoction of Śaramūlas with sugar and honey.
5. Decoction of Madhuyaṣṭhī, Śaramūla, Triphalā, Sitāvarikā with sugar and honey.
6. Decoction of Tṛṇa Pañcamūla drugs with sugar and honey.
7. Decoction of Śatāvarī, Prathakparṇī, Kulttha, and Badar with sugar and honey.
8. Juice of Tṛṇa Pañcamūla drugs with salt and ghṛta or with Rāsnā and Gokṣuru.
9. Milk medicated with Dusaka, Bṛahatī (both), Gokṣuru, Kuṭaja (both), Ārdraka, Yava, Darbha, Vṛkṣādanī, Balā and Pippalī with ghṛta is especially effective in raktaja mūtrakṛccha.

These recipes contain the drugs which are diuretic and astringent, by forceful flushing of urinary tract may wash out the infection, and relieve the symptom of mūtrakṛccha.

Mūtrāghāta or Mūtragraha

Mādhava is of opinion that when a person consumes rūkṣa (dry) articles and controls the urges of passing urine and stool, he may suffer from mūtrāghāta. It may be of 13 types, like—Vātakuṇḍala, aṣṭhīla, vātavasti, etc.[232]

Many texts of later period have mentioned a recipe for management of mutrāghāta in children. It contains the powdered Kaṇā (Pippalī), Ūṣaṇa (Marica), Elā (Laghu) and rock salt. This should be given with sugar-candy and honey.[233]

Śaiyyā-Mūtratā

Vangasena[234] has noticed the complaint of Śaiyyā-mūtratā and mentioned its management in his text. No etiology has been described by him. It may be considered as nocturnal enuresis as per description in modern texts. Nocturnal enuresis usually has no organic basis and is due to delayed maturation of bladder control or due to emotional factors. Organic disorders that may cause nocturnal enuresis include nocturnal epilepsy, urinary tract infection, D. mellitus, D. insipidus, obstructive uropathy, chronic renal failure etc. It is present in about 10-15% of otherwise normal 5 years old children and in about 1% of normal children at 15 years.

Management:

Vangasena has not mentioned any specific therapy for its management, except psychological therapy and a formal recipe.

1. The child is said to sit on his knees, at the place where he use to pass urine. He is asked to hold his finger of foot and then rice are offered to eat.
2. The clay, collected from the place of urination (of child) should be fried in Kāñjī and prescribed to the child with honey and ghṛta.

The use of this recipe should be very limited. In the light of modern knowledge it may be said that Vangasena was very right in his views. Because like his views modern science is also of similar view that this condition is benign and self-limiting, and steps should be taken to eliminate the emotional impact of the problem on child.

The following simple guidelines are described in modern paediatric texts, for management of the child with nocturnal enuresis:

1. Avoid ingestion of fluids after evening meal.
2. Void before retiring.
3. Rouse the child to void, before, the parent retires.
4. Counsel the parents to avoid emotional reactions.
5. Drug Therapy (Imipramine) should not be considered in children under 6 years of age and should not be used continuously after 8 weeks.

J. OTHER SYMPTOMS/DISORDERS

There are several many other symptoms or disorders which may manifest in child very commonly. These may also be chief characteristic features of many diseases of children, e.g., Jvara, Pāṇḍu, Kāmalā, etc. Kṛmi-roga was the common manifestation even in ancient period, which is also prevalent now-a-days in most of the tropical countries, including India. The texts, after Caraka Saṃhitā and Suśrutā Saṃhitā, have mentioned various recipes for the management of such common problems.

The description of these symptoms or disorders is general and applicable in both, child and adult. It appears not to be logical to discuss all the aspects, because this study is concerned only with the description, which is specifically mentioned for children. Therefore, only general concepts along with specific description (including treatment), related to children are recapitulated and discussed here.

Jvara (Pyrexia)

It is one of the most commonest symptoms of various disorders, affecting children. Most of the ancient scholars have described various general aspects of Jvara. Caraka opines that for jvara, involvement of deha, mana and indriya, is essential to feel santāpa.[235] Suśruta[236] has described 3 cardinal features of jvara:

(i) Blockade of sweating.

(ii) Sensation of heat in the body, and

(iii) Bodyache

Jvara may be classified into two groups (according to etiological factors—sahaja and āgantuja.

Sahaja jvarva arises from vitiation of doṣas, while āgantuja jvara may arise from four types of āgantuja (external) factors - abhicāra, abhighāta, abhiṣanga and abhiśāpa.

Caraka has described total 8 types of jvara. These are Vātaja, Pittaja, Kaphaja, Vātapittaja, Vāta-kaphaja, Pitta-kaphaja, Sannipātaja and Āgantuja. Sannipāta has been further sub-divided into 13 types.[237]

The jvara passes through four stages during its course-āmajvara (gradual increase in fever), pacyamāna jvara (high fever), pakva jvara (gradually becomes mild or stage of remission) and mukta jvara (feeling of lightness or afebrile stage).

Pothagenesis:

The doṣas, aggrevated with its causes afflicts āmāśaya, gets mixed up with agni, follows the course of rasa, which is the first product after the transformation of food; obstructs the channel of rasa and sweat, suppresses the activity of agni, extradicts the heat from the site of digestion (āmāśaya) and spreads it all over the body, causing jvara.[238]

Principles of Management:

During the stage of pūrva-rūpa, intake of light food or fasting is useful; because āmāśaya is the seat of the origin of this disease. Thereafter, depending upon the dosa involved and the therapeutic property, the patient should be administered decoction, drink, unction, oleation, fomentation, ointment, bath, emesis, purgation, āsthāpana (a type of enema), etc.[239]

Treatment specifically mentioned for children to cure the jvara (fever) is recapitulated here. The Kāśyapa Saṃhitā though mentioned a separate chapter on various aspects of treatment of fever, like nature of fever in newborns, its characters and dietetic regimen for kṣīrāda, kṣirānnāda and annāda children. But explanations of these concepts are unfortunately not available in the text due to missing of manuscript. This text contains description of management of 8 types of fever, in Khilasthāna,[240] however, Vranda is of opinion that the fever in children should be treated on the same principles as in adults. In Yoga Ratnasamuccaya, a long list of recipes for treatment of fever is given which is as follows:[241]

1. Paste of Rohiṇī mixed with fresh butter should be used orally as well as topically.
2. Application of mixture of ghṛta and maṇḍa over forehead, is effective.
3. Paste prepared with Kaṭurohiṇī and juice of Sahadevī, should be used orally, and topically; to get relief from all the types of fever.
4. Decoction of Kṣudrā, Śuṇṭhī, Guḍūcī and Pippalī.
5. Milk medicated with Aśvattha, etc. drugs.
6. Various religious measures, sacrifices (bali) and mantra therapy have been also claimed to be effective in getting relief from fever.

Recipes mentioned in Gada nigraha are:

1. Beverages (pānaka) prepared with Devadāru, Tagara, Madhuyaṣṭhī, Mañjiṣṭhā and sugar-candy; is especially effective in vātaja jvara.
2. Avaleha made of Lājā, Añjana, Vāṃsī, Madhuyaṣṭhī and sugar-candy should be offered to child suffering from fever of any origin.

Pāṇḍu (Paller or Anemia) & Kāmalā (Jaundice)

In ancient texts these two conditions are described together. Most of the Āyurvedic texts consider that Kāmalā is an advance stage of Pāṇḍu. Line of treatment of both these conditions is also similar.

(A) Pāṇḍu (Pallor or Anemia)

The person who appears Pāṇḍura (pallor), is said to suffer from Pāṇḍu. The main cause of pallorness is deficient haemoglobin contents of blood, and the condition is known as anemia.

Caraka has described 5 types of Pāṇḍu—vātika, paittika, kaphaja, sannipātika and mṛttikā bhakṣaṇajanya.[242]

Etiopathogenesis:

By intake of alkaline, sour, saltish, too hot, incompatible and unsuitable food; excessive use of niṣpāva, black gram oil cake, tila and oil; day sleep; exercise etc. during digestion of food; suppression of natural urges; various psychological factors like—anxiety, fear, anger and grief; the pitta is aggravated.

The aggravated pitta is propelled by vāyu, from heart into ten arteries, which spread it in the whole body. This pitta located in the space between tvaka (skin) and māṃsa (muscle) affect kapha, vāta, rakta, tvacā and māṃsa and thereby produces various shades of colours like pale, yellow, deep yellow or green, in skin.[243]

Common causes which may manifest anemia are blood loss, nutritional defects, infection, haemolysis, defective red cell production and other serious blood diseases.

General Features:

The main features of this disorder is pāṇḍutva. The premonitory symptoms are—Palpitation, roughness, absence of sweat and exhaustion. The specific features of pānḍu depends upon the associated vitiated doṣa.[244]

(B) Kāmalā (Jaundice)

The patient of pāṇḍu roga when excessively and regularly consumes the articles increasing pitta, his pitta gets vitiated more and affect rakta (blood) and māṃsa (muscle) producing Kāmalā.

The eyes, skin and nails become similar, to colour of Haridrā. Urine and stool becomes yellowish with some blood. The colour of patient become similar to frog of rainy season.[245]

Reference of Kāmalā are even in Vedas.[246]

Caraka has described its two types: Koṣṭhāśrita and Śākhāśrita.[247]

It may be considered as jaundice or hyperbilirubinemia, according to modern knowledge. It is an important manifestation of hepatic dysfunction that may result from failure of bilirubin uptake into the liver cell, conjugation with glucoronide, transport within the hepatocyte, or excretion across canaliculi. Jaundice may also reflect the normal functional immaturity of the developing infants.

Principles of Management of Pāṇḍu and Kāmalā:

Management of these two conditions is most of the time described together. The patient of Pāṇḍu roga after unction, should be subjected to emesis and purgation, while that of Kāmalā with comparatively mild purgation with bitter drugs. After this, both types of cases should be managed with wholesome diet such as old śāli rice, barley and wheat with soup of green gram, lentiles or meat soup of wild animals and birds. Medicaments should be administered according to doṣa and as specific to the disorder.[248]

Mṛttikā-bhakṣaṇa-janya pāṇḍu is very common in children. Therefore, for treating such cases, first of all ingested clay should be eliminated by administering evacuation according to strength. There after when the body gets cleaned, the strength promoting ghṛta should be administered. Caraka has given an other alternative for the patients who does not desist from earth eating. These cases should provide clay, after impregnated with the drugs which destroy its harmful effect, such as Viḍanga, Elā, Ativiṣā, Nimba leaves, Pāṭhā, Brahatī (fruits), Kaṭurohiṇī, Indrayava or Mūrvā.[249]

It has been considered by modern scientists that on consuming clay, the various ova and cysts of parasites (especially, Ankylostoma dudenale) are infested, which really produces anemia due to sucking the blood of the person from its intestinal mucosa. The drugs prescribed for purification of clay are kṛmighna which keeps it free from worms.

The concept of phototherapy for treatment of Kāmalā has come from Vedas and now-a-days it is the only method for management of neo-natal jaundice.

Specific recipes:

Some recipes have been mentioned by ancient texts which are useful in curing the pāṇḍu roga in children.

1. Cow's urine mixed with powdered Mūrvā, Dhātakī, Haridrā and honey.
2. Ghṛta medicated with Triphalā and Bhrngarāja.[250]
3. Powdered Haridrā, Devadāru, Saralā, Karkataṣrangī, Brahatī (both), Praśniparṇī, Śatapuṣpā with honey and ghṛta is effective in treating pāṇḍu.[251]

The above mentioned recipes do not contain any iron preparation, which is very essential to replace the loss. Here the concepts of ancient scholars are basically different from modern scientists.

Ancient idea is that by using dīpana, pācana therapy (as mentioned above) improve the pācakāgni and dhātvāgni resulting in better absorption and assimilation of iron from the diet consumed by the child.

Kṛimis

Though references of kṛimis are found in different diseases like Pāṇḍu, Grahaṇī, Kuṣṭha, Yakṣamā, as one of the causative factor but most of the texts have described it as a separate disease entity. Vedas have ample references of kṛimis. The description includes names, their morphological features and treatment. Atharva veda mentions the infestation of children from Krimis.[252] Most of the Āyurvedic texts have given classification, features, causative factors and diseases produced by kṛimis.

Classification:

Āyurvedic texts[253] have described 20 varieties of kṛimis as mentioned in the following Table 41.

Table 41: Types of krimis described in various Āyurvedic texts

Types	*Names described in Āyurvedic texts*		
	C.S.	*S.S.*	*A.S.; A.H.*
External	Yūkā	-	Yūka
	Pipīlikā	-	Likṣā
Internal:			
a. Raktaja	Keśāda	Keśāda	Keśāda
	Lomāda	Lomāda	Loma vidhva-ṃsaka
	Loma dvīpa	Dantāda	Loma dvīpa
	Saurasa	Kikkisa	Saurasa
	Audumbara	Kuṣṭhaja	Audumbara
	Jantumata	Parisarpa	Jantumata
b. Kaphaja	Āntrāda	Mahāpuṣpa	Āntrāda
	Udarāda	Pralūna	Udarāda
	Hṛdaya para (7)	Dāruṇa(6)	Hṛdaya para(7)
	Caru	Cipita	Curu
	Darbhapuṣpa	Darbhapuṣpa	Darbhapuṣpa
	Saugandhika	-	Saugandhika
	Mahāguda	-	Mahāguda
c. Purisaja	Kakeruka	Ajava	Kakeruka
	Makeruka	Vijavā	Makeruka
	Leliha	Kipyā	Lelihya
	Saśūlaka	Cipya	Saśūlaka
	Sausurāda	Gaṇḍūpada	Sausurāda
		Curu	
		Dvimukha	

Etiological Factors, External Features and Clinical Manifestations

(a) *Vāhya (external) kṛimis*—These are similar to the shape and colour of moles (tila) appeared from mala and are mostly found in hairs and cloths. These are minute in appearance, having number of feet (polypoda). Manifest with eruption, boils, enlargement of glands and itching.[254]

(b) *Ābhyantara (internal) Kṛimis*—Generally most of the ābhyantara kṛimis develop due to routine habit of consumption of food even in indigestion, excessive use of sweet and sour articles and jaggery, sleep in day and lack of exercise.

These manifest with fever, discolouration, pain, cardiac disorders, weakness of body parts, confusion, anorexia and diarrhoea.[255]

Principles of Treatment:

In Atharva Veda sun rays are considered to kill the kṛimis.[256] Now-a-days it is well proved that sun rays contain various specific rays like ultra violet, etc., which have the properties to kill the bacterias.

Caraka[257] has given certain principles for treating the patient of Kṛīmis. These are: Saṃśodhana, Kṛimi apakarṣaṇa and Prakriti vighāta.

1. Saṃśodhana—Initially Kṛimis are stimulated by snehana, svedana and diet favourable from them. Then Saṃśodhana is to be done by āsthāpana, vamana and virecana.

   For children use of Kaṭu, Tikta and Rukṣa articles; cow's urine and rock salt are prescribed for snehana and svedana.

An other method for svedana is also advised by Kaśyapa. For this purpose kaṭu-taila and rock salt are applied in the rectum, then svedana is performed by a finger (after rubbing to produce heat).

After milk medicated with various drugs has been considered congenial.

For external kṛimis, bath mentioned for treatment of vṛṇa (in Kaśyapa Saṃhitā) should be applied.

In case of very small children (infants) all the purificatory (saṃśodhana) measures should be performed on dhātrī.[258]

2. Kṛimi aparkarṣaṇa—Caraka has described several methods for extracting the kṛimis. These are—removal by hand, by use of drugs, prakṛtivighāta (change in environment), nidāna parivarjana (removal of cause).[259]

Specific Recipes for Children Suffering from Kṛimi:

For treatment of kṛimis, mostly those drugs are used which are kaṭu, tikta, kaṣāya, kṣāra and ūṣṇa.

Kaśyapa has advised to use Vidanga ghṛta. It should be administered with sugar.[260] Anti-helmenthic property of Viḍanga is well proved today.

K. BĀLA GRAHAS

The graha rogas have separate entity from other general disorders, as their etiological factors, features and managements are entirely different. There is common belief that certain uncommon or unidentified factor, may exclusively affect to children.

The word 'Graha' means to seize or grasp.[261] Thus grahas are said to be a class of evil demons supposed to capture or affect the child producing various features. In Mahābhārata, it has been described very clearly that these bāla grahas affect the children up to the age of 16 years.[262]

The concept of grahas exist right from Vedic period. In Atharva Veda, the word Grahī appears, which is commented by Sāyaṇa as Rākṣasī, and is said to attack the children.[263]

Kauśika Sūtra has written a prayer to get rid of grāhi.[264] Ṛg Veda and Atharva Veda have described demons attacking the foetus and neonates.[265]

The description of Skanda Bhaiṣajya, Jambha and treatment of various grahas are found in Kauśika Sūtra.[266] Similarly some other gṛhya-sūtras havẹ also described the management of nine grahas.[267]

Mahābhārata has included extensive description of bāla grahas,[268] and mentioned morphology and features of Skanda, Skandāpasmāra, Śakunī, Pūtanā, Śītapūtanā, Revatī and Mukhamaṇḍikā,[269]

Varāhamihira has mentioned the effect and worship of nine grahas (planets), which are different from grahas mentioned by other scholars. However, those are also said to influence the body.

In Agni Purāṇa, the term 'grahī' has been used for grahas, as these are considered as female grahas. These affect the child from very first day of his life, till 17 years of age. On this basis these grahas have been classified according to days (10), months (12), and years (16). Thus the total number of grahas, affecting the children (birth to 17 years) become 38. Bāla Tantra compiled by Vaidya Kalyāṇa has given quite similar description.

Mārkaṇḍeya Purāṇa[270] has described about 16 demons appeared from Nirmasti, wife of Dusaha (demon). Out of these 8 are male and 8 are female. These may affect to child as well as fetus, developing in womb. Concept of Jātihariṇī also might have come from Kaśyapa Saṃhitā.

In Āyurvedic texts various aspects of bāla-grahas have been discussed in detail. Caraka Saṃhitā[271] has no direct reference of grahas, however, influence of 'Deva' are supposed to cause various disorders like grahas and appear with indifferent etilogy with typical features, without proper correlation with vitiation of doṣas. Suśruta has given much importance of bāla grahas and given elaborative account on this aspect, including predisposing factors, mode of seizure, manifestations and management of individual grahas. These are 9 in number, and named as—Skanda, Skandāpasmāra, Śakunī, Revatī, Pūtanā, Andhapūtanā, Śītapūtanā, Mukhamaṇḍikā and Naigmeṣa.[272] Vāgbhaṭa has added 3 more grahas. Thus the total number become 12, which have been classified as male and female grahas. Male grahas are five—Skanda, Viśākha, Meṣa, Śvagraha, Pitragraha; while female are seven—Śakunī, Pūtanā, Śītapūtanā, Adraṣṭi Pūtanā (Andha Pūtanā), Mukhamaṇḍikā, Revatī and Śuṣka Revatī.[273]

In Kaśyapa Saṃhitā, references of bāla grahas are found at three different places:

(i) In Sūtra sthāna, the available description is incomplete (due to missing of manuscript), yet vitiation of dhātrī milk with Śakunī, Skanda, Saṣṭhī and Pūtanā have been mentioned. Kaśyapa, has given first time this concept of vitiation of breast milk through influence of grahas. On consuming such milk the child may present with various features of graha.[274]

(ii) Features of manifestation and management of various grahas, like Skanda, Skandāpasmāra, Pitraskanda, Puṇḍarīka, Revatī, Śuṣkarevatī, Śakunī, Mukhamaṇḍikā, Pūtanā and Naigmeṣa, have been described in Indriyasthāna[275].

(iii) While describing treatment of bāla grahas, Kaśyapa has mentioned about Revatī, Pūtanā, Andhapūtanā, Śītapūtanā, Kaṭpūtanā and Mukharcikā (Mukhamaṇḍikā).[276]

Pūtanā has been mentioned with its 20 names; various types of 'Jātihāriṇīs' have been described, affecting the growing fetus and neonates.[277] Probably the concept of Jātihāriṇī came from Vedas. Ṛg Veda and Atharva Veda have described various Kṛimis and demons, which were supposed to attack the fetus and neonate.[278]

Kalyāṇa Kāraka (a treatise of Jain period), has discussed bāla-grahas under 'Bhūta Tantrādhikāra.' Though the description is similar to Suśruta Saṃhitā and Aṣṭānga Saṃgraha and numbers are also nine, yet names of certain grahas have been changed like, Kinnara, Anupūtanā, Piśāca and Rākṣasa grahas, Skanda, Andhapūtanā, Mukhamaṇḍikā and Naigmeṣa; respectively. No use of 'bali' has been mentioned for the treatment of bāla-grahas. Probably this was due to effect of religious principles of Jains i.e., Ahiṃsā.[279]

Cakradatta contains full description of 'Kumāra-Tantra' of Rāvaṇa, in which 12 bāla-grahas are mentioned. Hārīta has described only one Strīgraha—Pūtanā, with its 8 types—Lohitā, Revatī, Vyāsī (dvānkṣī), Kumārī, Śakunī, Śivā, Urdhvakeśī and Senā. These attack to the child on the day, month and year in the same order.[280]

Table 42: Names of various bāla-grahas (as described in different Āyurvedic texts)

CS	*SS*	*KS*	*AS/AH*	*KK*	*KT(R)*	*HS*
No. innumerable	*(9)*	-	*(12)*			
'Deva'	Skanda	Skanda	Skanda	Kinnara	Nandā	Pūtanā
	Skandāpasmāra	Skandāpasmāra	Viśākha	Skanda	-	(8 types)
	Śakunī	Śakunī	Śakunī	Śakunī	Śakunikā	Lohitā
	Pūtanā	Pūtanā	Pūtanā	Pūtanā	Pūtanā	Revatī
	Andhapūtanā	Andhapūtanā	Adrṣṭipūtanā	Anupūtanā		Vayasi
	Śītapūtanā	Śītapūtanā	Śītapūtanā	Śītapūtanā	-	Kumārī
	Mukhamaṇḍikā	Mukharcikā	Mukhamaṇḍikā	Piśāca	Mukha	Śakuni, Śivā
	Naigmeṣa	Naigmeṣa	Meṣa	Rākṣas	-	Ūrdhvakeśī
	Revatī	Revatī	Revatī	Revatī		Senā
		Śuṣkarevatī	Śuṣkarevatī	Śuṣkarevatī		
		Pitṛskanda	Pitṛgraha	-		
		Saṣṭhī	Śvagraha	-		
		Puṇḍarīka	-	-		
		Kaṭputanā	-	Kaṭpūtanā		
		Jātahāriṇīs	-	Āryaka		
		Revatī		Sūtikā		
		(With 20 names)		Pillipiccikā		
				Kamuka		
				Sunandā		
				Nirita		

ETIO-PATHOGENESIS OF BĀLA-GRAHA

The disorders produced by influence of Grahas are not primarily due to vitiation of doṣas but are āgantuja (external) in nature. The grahas are syndromes, caused by demons and may be infectious in nature. Kaśyapa opined clearly that these can be seen only by divine eyes.[281] It clears that these grahas may be like micro-organisms. Children are mostly affected by grahas, because they are dependent on others, therefore, are unable to maintain proper hygiene by themselves. Secondly, children are deficient in immunity thus more susceptible for various influences including bāla grahas.

Suśruta has imagined very intelligently that how these grahas, enter in the body. He opines that grahas enter the body unperceived like an image in a mirror or heat of sun-rays by a lense or like the soul entering the body.[282]

Suśruta has further given a list of conditions in which graha attacks the child:[283]

1. Rules of conduct and hygiene are not followed by mother/nurse.

2. The child is fearful due to threatening, beating or frightened.

3. The priest, saints, teachers and guests are not respected.

4. Dhātrī or mother is indulged excessively in eating, sex, sleep, exercise, harmful activities and other unreligious conducts.

5. The child or mother take food in unclean and broken vessels.

6. The child is carried to lonely and inauspicious places.

Vāgbhaṭa has described the purpose for which graha attacks. These are to cause evil, to get themselves worshipped, and to get their sexual passions pacified.[284]

The first group gives more or less similar to infective disorders while the second and third presents a derangement in behaviours. However, the bāla grahas seem to attack the child only to cause some evil.

GENERAL SYMPTOMS IN A CHILD AFFECTED WITH BĀLA-GRAHAS

The symptoms appearing in a child due to affection of bāla-graha, may depend upon the infliction of that particular graha.

Various symptoms may be classified as follows (Table 43).

Table 43: Showing various symptoms of Bāla-Grahas[285]

	Symptoms in child
1. General symptoms	Fever, irritability, excessive crying yawning, shouts, bites lips, clenches teeth, clenches fists, injures himself or the mother with the nails or teeth, refusal to take feeds, emaciation, excessive salivation, excessive lacrimation, rubs his eyes, ears and nose, miserable look, eyes become red, etc.
2. Central Nervous System	
(a) Psychological	Fear, pulls his hairs, laughs alone without any reason, becomes cruel.
(b) Organic	Vacant stare, unconsciousness, drowsiness, giddiness, irritability, hypotonia, rolling of eye-balls, jerky movements of head, twitching of eyelids and facial muscles, tremors, defective posture, dribling of saliva (due to facial palsy), change in voice and speech, incontinence of urine and stool, fainting, etc.
3. Gastro-intestinal symptoms	Diarrhoea, distension, vomiting thirst, constipation, stomatitis, etc.
4. Respiratory symptoms	Cough, hiccup, grunting respiration, etc.
5. Skin	Change in colour of skin, blisters urticaria, prominent veins over skin of abdomen, etc.
6. Smell of body	The child may emit fishy, bed bug like, fleshy or bloody, etc. smell according to influence of particular grahas.

DESCRIPTION OF INDIVIDUAL GRAHAS

The grahas are said to be very minute, therefore, cannot be seen by ordinary persons with their nacked eyes. Their presence should be considered only by the features appeared in the child due to their attack. However, the scholars like Suśruta and Vāgbhaṭa have personified the grahas. The Mahābhārata has also mentioned the morphological features (imaginary) of various grahas like, Skanda, Skandāpasmāra, Śakunī, Putanā, Śītapūtanā, Revatī. and Mukhamaṇḍikā. The morphological characters of grahas may be helpful in planning the treatment (daiva vyapāṣraya cikitsā).

Symptoms of attack are also described in detail by Suśruta and Vāgbhaṭa. On the basis of those symptoms all the graha rogas (syndromes) may be kept parallel to certain diseases, described in modern medicine (as mentioned in Table 57).

Skanda Graha

Skanda graha has been considered the chief of grahas; bearing golden crown, garland of red flowers, red cloths and his body is smeared with red sandalwood paste, and of charming personality. Varāhamihira has also described the shape of Skanda.[286]

Symptoms of Attack

According to description of Suśruta,[287] Skanda graha present the features of facial palsy. The following Table 44 may clear the picture.

Table 44 : Showing features of Skanda graha (described by Suśruta) and their correlation with facial palsy.

Features of Skanda graha	*Facial palsy*
1. Inflammation of eyes	+
2. The child appears restless	+
3. Deviation of angle of mouth	+
4. There is absent or excessive movement of one eye lid	+
5. Refusal to suck	+
6. The child likes to close his eyes	+
7. Less weeping	+
8. Fists become tight	±
9. Usual complaint of constipation	-
10. The child emits the smell of blood	-

Considering the views of Vāgbhata,[288] Skanda graha may be considered as polio-encephalitis with the following features (Table 45).

Table 45: Features of Skanda graha (as described by Vāgbhaṭa) and their correlation with the features of polio-encephalitis

Skanda Graha	*Polio-encephalitis*
1. Excessive lacrimation from one eye	+
2. Half side of body become paralysed (monoplagia)	+
3. Recurrent convulsions	+
4. The body becomes stiff	+
5. Excessive sweating	±
6. Dropping of neck	+

7.	The child looks frightened, restless and bits (his lips)	+
8.	Deviation of mouth and excessive salivation	+
9.	Upwards deviated eyes	+
10.	Unvoluntary movements of one eye, eye brows and face	±
11.	Tights his fists	+
12.	Flushing of face	±
13.	Constipation	+

Vāgbhaṭa has considered that this graha is very fatal. The affected child may die, if survives he becomes disabled.

The above description indicates that observation of this disease, made by Suśruta is related to only facial involvement, while Vāgbhaṭa has taken the problem very seriously. The features of facial palsy (as described by Suśruta) are few among the features, presenting the total picture of the disease, i.e., encephalitic form of polio. Thus Skanda graha may be very well correlated with polio-encephalitis.

Skandāpasmāra (Viśākha)

It has been also described with the name of Viśākha. Appearance is bright like fire (agni) and is beloved friend of Skanda.[289]

Symptoms of Attack:[290]

The Skandāpasmāra may be considered as a convulsive disorder of childhood period. The most common cause of cunvulsion may be epilepsy. The following features of Skandāpasmāra are in favour of seizure (Table 46).

Table 46: Features of Skandāpasmāra and their correlation with seizures

Skandāpasmāra	*Epilepsy*
1. Recurrent loss of consciousness with irregular movements of limbs and froathing from mouth.	+
2. The child plucks his hair and may bite his tongue or nipples of his mother.	+
3. The child may pass urine and stool involuntarily	+
4. Yawning may be associated with typical sound (cry).	+
5. Associated features:	
(i) Fever	+
(ii) awakening in night	-
(iii) smell of body like pus and blood.	-

Presence of convulsion may be due to fever. In childhood period the common cause of convulsion may be high fever, and known as febrile convulsion. These febrile convulsions are unusual before the age of 6 months, and they should not be diagnosed after the age of 5 years. The peak age incidence is 18 months. These children may suffer from epilepsy, in later life.

Meṣa Graha (Naigameṣa)

Meṣa is also known as Naigameṣa. His face is like goat with moving eye brows and eye-balls. He can acquire the shape, according to his desire.[291]

Symptoms of Attack:

The features of seizure by meṣa graha[292] are shown in Table 47.

Table 47: Features of Meṣa Graha

Meṣa Graha	*Meningitis*
1. Stiffness of body, stooping in the middle	+
2. Loss of consciousness with irregular movements of limbs, clinching of fists and bits his lips.	+
3. Upward deviated look	+
4. Fever (continuous type)	+
5. Associated features—hiccough, cough, diarrhoea	±
6. Swelling of one eye	-
7. The child emits the smell of goat	-

The Meṣa graha has very much resemblance with meningitis or features of meningial irritation.

With the following cardinal features, Meṣa graha may be considered as meningitis or meningism.

1. Presence of fever.
2. Stiffness of body, especially of neck.
3. Convulsions.
4. Loss of consciousness (coma).

Pūtanā Graha

Pūtanā is a she-demon and looks dirty, fearful, black complexion with bad smell. She likes to live in broken houses.[293]

Features of Attack:[294]

Table - 48 : Features of Pūtanā graha

Pūtanā graha	*Diarrhoea 8 dehydration 8 electrolyte imbalance*
1. Diarrhoea and vomiting	+
2. Body appears relaxed	+
3. The child likes to drink much water	+
4. Associated Symptoms:	
- retention of urine	+
- distension of abdomen	+
- hiccough, etc.	-

All these above features are of gastro-enteritis with dehydration and electrolyte imbalance (hypopotassaemia). The child likes to drink much water, due to dehydration. Flaccidity of body parts and distension of abdomen, clearly indicates towards associated hypopotassaemia.

Śītapūtanā

Śītapūtanā likes to live by the side of water reservoirs and likes to eat mudga, rice, wine and blood.[295]

Features of Attack:[296]

Features of attack of Śītapūtanā are discussed in the following Table 49.

Table 49: Features of Śītapūtana

Śītapūtanā graha	*Diarrhoea & dehydration & hyponaetrimia*
1. Diarrhoea and thirst	+
2. The child shivers repeatedly	+
3. Gurgling sounds in abdomen	±
4. The body is warm on one side while cool on the other.	±
5. The child emits smell like fat	-

The features mentioned for attack of Śītapūtanā may be considered as diarrhoea with dehydration and hyponaetrimia.

Andhapūtanā

Andhapūtanā is of terrifying and brown in appearance. She wears sofronin garments and her head is bald. She is also known as Drṣṭipūtanā.[297] In Mahābhārata, she has been said to affect the fetus.

Features of Attack:[298]

Features of attack of Andhapūtanā are summarised in the following Table 50.

Table 50: Features of attack of Andhapūtanā

Andhapūtanā	*Diarrhoea 8 Vit. A deficiency*
1. The child suffers from diarrhoea, vomiting, fever, cough, etc.	+
2. Child does not like food	+
3. Emaciation and discolouration of body.	+
4. Gradual loss of vision and various other eye complications	+
5. The child becomes irritable with sharp voice.	±

With these above features it may be concluded that Andha-pūtanā is a condition of chronic diarrhoea associated with Vitamin A deficiency. Due to diarrhoea, etc. complaints, the child does not like food and he gradually becomes emaciated, which further leads to develop poor absorption capacity. Children develop Vit. A deficiency, may manifest the symptoms of Vit. A deficiency when it is not adequately taken or poorly absorbed. Along with defective vision, Vit. A deficiency is also responsible for poor resistance power, leading to various symptoms like cough, fever and changes in skin, etc.

Pitṛgraha

Pitṛgraha has been mentioned by Vāgbhaṭa and considered that this graha is superior to all other grahas. It resides near the roots of trees.[299]

Features of Attack:[300]

The features appeared due to attack of Pitṛgraha are similar to respiratory infection with parenteral diarrhoea.

Table 51: Features of Pitṛgraha in comparison with respiratory infections with parenteral diarrhoea

Pitṛgraha	*Respiratory infection & parent. diarrhoea*
1. Fever, cough, diarrhoea and vomiting	+
2. Excessive thirst	+
3. Convulsions	+
4. Emaciation and discolouration of body	±
5. The child looks frightened and weeps suddenly	±
6. Excessive lacrimation	-
7. The child emits the smell of dead body	-

The above features suggest that Pitṛgraha may be a condition of respiratory infection with parental diarrhoea.

Śvagraha

The word 'śva' may be referred for a dog (śvāna), thus this graha may be said as dog demon. It has been created by Lord Śiva and Pārvatī, for protection of Kārtikeya. This graha has been mentioned by Vāgbhaṭa.[301]

Symptoms of Attack:

The child may present with following features, seized by Śwagraha.

Table 52: Features of attack of Śwagraha

Śwagraha		*Rabies*
1.	The child develop tremors with sweating, closing of eyelids and erection of hairs (romaharṣa)	+
2.	He may bite his tongue	+
3.	The posture become opisthotonos	+
4.	Typical cry or sound like barking of dog	+
5.	The child runs	±
6.	Body emits the faecal smell	-

The child affected with Śvagraha presents the features which are very close to rabies, a very fatal disease transmitted to human by inoculation of the infected saliva of an animal (usually dog).

The features in favour are—rigidity and spasms of muscles, typical cry or sound due to spasm of pharynx and running of the child.

Revatī Graha

Revatī is a dark complexioned demon which wears the clothes of various colours and is decorated with a typical type of garlands and smeared with paste of sandal wood. She is with oscillating ear rings.[303]

Suśruta has mentioned that Revatī may be also known as Lamba, Karāla, Vinitā, Bahuputrikā and Śuṣka Revatī. Kaśyapa has given 20 synonyms of it, while in Mahābhārata, she has been said Aditi and Raivata.

Symptoms of Attack:[304]

The features appeared due to seizure of Revatī graha are mentioned in the Table 53.

Table 53: Features of attack of Revatī

Revatī Graha	*Diarrhoea & anemia & Vit. B Complex deficiency*
1. The mouth becomes red	-
2. Loose stools are greenish	+
3. The associated features:	
(i) Fever	±
(ii) Stomatitis	+
(iii) Pain	±
(iv) Discolouration	+
4. The child usually rubs the eyes, ears and nose	-
5. Becomes emaciated and face appear emaciated.	±

The features of Revatī graha presents with the features of diarrhoea with emaciation and anemia. The stomatitis may be due to associated deficiency of vitamins B complex group.

Śuṣka Revatī

Vāgbhaṭa[305] has mentioned in detail about this graha while Suśruta has included it in the Revatī and mentioned as a synonym of Revati.

Symptoms of Attack:[306]

The child presents with the following features (Table 54)

Table 54: Features of attack of Śuṣka Revatī.

Śuṣka Revatī	*Koch's abdomen*
1. The child passes loose greenish stools, sometime of variegated colour.	+
2. The abdomen presents nodular feelings and appearance of prominent veins over abdomen	+
3. The child gradually becomes emaciated	+
4. Associated features:	
(i) fall of hair	+
(ii) Aversion from food	+
(iii) Weak voice	+
(iv) Discolouration	+
(v) Excessive cry	±
5. Emits the smell of eagle	-

The features of Śuṣka Revatī are suggestive of abdominal tuberculosis (Koch's abdomen). The characteristic features in favour are—nodular feeling in abdomen, loose stools of various colours and progressive emaciation. Though there is mild to moderate pyrexia associated with Koch's abdomen, however, it may not present as an specific features in chronic stage probably due to loss of immunity, therefore may not described by Vāgbhaṭa.

Śakunī Graha

Śakunī demon remains decorated with ornaments, her eyes are brown with huge body and large belly. She is down looking with sharp beak and ugly face. Her ears are large and cone shaped. She likes to wander in sky.[307]

Symptoms of Attack:[308]

The child seized by Śakunī graha may have following characteristics (Table 55).

Table 55: Showing features of Śakunī graha and comparison with Impetigol

Śakunī graha	*Impetigo*
1. The child looks frightened with flexed body parts.	+
2. Body is full of blisters with burning pain and inflammation.	+
3. Oozing blisters ultimately form ulcer	+
4. Constitutional symptoms:	+
1. Fever	+
2. Diarrhoea	±
5. The child emits the smell like Śakunī (a bird)	±

The above features of Śakunī graha are more near to Impetigo, which is an acute infection caused by staphylococcus organism and most commonly affect to newborns.

Mukhamaṇḍikā Graha

Mukhamaṇḍikā[309] is a charming demon decorated with ornaments. She can change her shape as per her desire and mostly resides in cowsheds. Its two synonyms—Subhagā and Kāmācāriṇī are described in Mahābhārata.

Symptoms of Attack:[310]

The child may have following features, seized by Mukhamaṇḍikā.

Table 56: Features of Mukhamaṇḍikā and its correlation with Indian childhood cirrhosis

Mukhamaṇḍikā	*Indian childhood cirrhosis*
1. Altered appetite	+
2. Abdomen appears full of blackish or bluish veins.	+
3. The child looks dull.	+
4. The hands, foot and face of child appear beautiful.	+
5. May suffer from fever.	±
6. Looks irritable.	+
7. Emits the smell of urine.	±

The features of the child, seized by Mukhamaṇḍikā graha resemble the picture of Indian Childhood Cirrhosis. The specific points in favour are—irritability, alterned appetite, fever and prominent abdominal veins. The beautiful shiny appearance of the child may be due to generalised oedema. In children with impending liver cell failure, a peculiar garlic odour is present, which may be described in ancient texts as smell of urine.

On the basis of presenting symptoms, the syndromes of bāla grahas may be classified into four groups. These may be also correlated with various disease entities, described in present day literatures of medicine. The description is summarized in the following Table 57.

Table 57: Classification of Bāla Grahas and their parallel diseases

Group based presenting symptoms	*Graha*	*Diseases equivalent*
1. Grahas presenting with neurological symptoms	Skanda	Polioencephalitis
	Skandā-pasmāra	Convulsive disorders (Epilepsy)
	Meṣa	Meningitis
	Śvagraha	Rabies
2. Grahas presenting with diarrhoea	Pitṛgraha	Resp. inf. & parent diarrhoea
	Pūtanā	Diar. & dehy. & hypokalemia
	Śītapūtanā	Diar. & dehy. & hypocalcemia
	Andhapūtanā	Diar. & dehy. & Vit. A deficiency.
	Revatī	Diar. & dehy. & Anemia & Vit. B. complex def.
3. Grahas presenting with prominent veins over abdominal wall	Śuṣkarevatī	Koch's abdomen
	Mukhamaṇḍikā	Indian Childhood Cirrhosis
4. Grahas presenting eruptions on skin.	Śakunī	Impetigo

Description of Graha (Grahī) in Agni Purāṇa

Agni Purāṇa has given a long list of grahīs affecting the child, from first day of his birth upto 17 years. The following Table provide the period of attack, name of grahī, along with the features, caused by them.[311]

Table 58: Showing period of attack, names and features appeared due to seizure of grahīs (described in Agni Purāṇa)

Period of attack	*Name*	*Features of attack*
DAY		
1st day of birth	Pāpinī	Excitement, refusal to feed
2nd day	Bhīṣaṇī	Cough, tremors
3rd day	Ghaṇṭālī	Excessive cry, refusal to suck
4th day	Kākolī	Excitement, excessive cry, froathing from mouth
5th day	Hansādhikā	Yawning, difficulty in respiration and tightening of fists
6th day	Faṭkārī	Unconscious, convulsions, some times excessive cry
7th day	Mukta keśī	Emits foul smell, yawning, excessive cry
8th day	Ṣridanḍī	Looks around, excessive movement of tongue, cough
9th day	Ūrdhva grahi	Excitement, difficulty in respiration
10th day	Rodanī	Excessive cry, body becomes bluish
MONTH		
1st month	Pūtanā	Cries like crow, deep respiration and emits smell of urine.
2nd month	Mukuṭā	Body becomes yellowish and cold, vomiting, running nose.
3rd month	Gomukhī	Sleepiness, passes urine and stool very frequently, cry.
4th month	Pingalā	Progressive emaciation, very fatal
5th month	Lalanā	Flaccid appearance, dryness of mouth, yellow colouration of body and excessive flatulence.
6th month	Pankajā	Cry and change in voice.
7th month	Nirahara	Suffers from dental disorders.
8th month	Yamunā	Boils on body and emaciation.

9th month	Kumbha karṇī	Fever, vomiting, cry
10th month	Tāpasī	Refusal to feed
11th month	Rākṣasī	Diseases of eyes.
12th month	Cancalā	Looks frightened.
YEARS		
2nd year	Yātanā	Cry.
3rd year	Rodanī	Weeping, shivering and urine with blood.
4th year	Cataka	Fever and pain in all body parts.
5th year	Cancalā	Flaccid extremities, fever, etc.
6th year	Dhavanī	Emaciation, pain in all body parts.
7th year	Yamunā	Vomiting, increased frequency of urination etc.
8th year	Jātavedā	Refusal to feed, cry.
9th year	Kalā	Tremors in arms, looks frightened, etc.
10th year	Kālahaṃsī	Fever, burning and emaciation
11th year	Devadūtī	Speaks hard.
12th year	Bālikā	Respiratory disorders.
13th year	Vāyavī	Diseases of mouth
14th year	Yakṣiṇī	Fever, burning and pain.
15th year	Muṇḍikā	Bleeding disorders.
16th year	Vānarī	Constant fever, sleep and usually fell down on ground (due to weakness).
17th year	Gandhavatī	Excitement, cries excessively.

Jātihāriṇī

Kaśyapa has given an unique concept of Jātihāriṇī.[312] This is also known as Revatī, Pilipicchikā, Raudrī and Vāruṇī and affect the women during her various stages, i.e., menstruation, pregnancy, etc. It also destructs the fetus and child. Jātihāriṇīs usually affect by not observing or following the rules of hygiene, diet and general mode of life by wife and husband both.

These may be classified in two ways—on the basis of prognosis and mode of transmission.

On the basis of prognosis these may be Sādhya (curable), Yāpya (easily relapcable), and Asādhya (incurable); while on the basis of mode of transmission these are Daivī (divine), Mānuṣī (human) and Tiraścīna (other living organisms, i.e., Śakunī, Catuṣpādī, Sarpa, Mātsī and Vanaspatī).

Kaśyapa has given a detailed account of various Jātihāriṇīs including their features and management.

On the basis of specific symptoms, these Jātihariṇīs may be correlated with various conditions. In this regard the description given by Prof. Tewari (Āyurvedīya Prasūti Tantra, Part I) appears more appropriate, which is as follows:

Table 59: Various Jātihāriṇīs and their equivalent diseases/conditions

Jātihāriṇīs	*Equivalent probable disease/condition*
1. Śuṣka-Revatī	Delayed menarche due to nutritional disorders.
2. Kaṭambharā	Primary amenorrhoea due to nutritional deficiency without influencing longevity.
3. Puṣpaghnī	Anovular menstruation associated with hirsutism
4. Vikuṭā	Irregularly irregular menstrual cycle.
5. Pariśrutā	Excessive vaginal discharges (leucorrhoea)
6. Aṇḍaghnī	Abortion of embryo (blastocystic stage)
7. Durdharā	Abortion during first trimester
8. Kālarātri	Premature delivery associated with death of neonate
9. Mohinī	Abortion due to diseases of mother.
10. Stambhanī	Absence of quickening or stillness of fetus.
11. Krośanā	Pregnancy disorders (toxaemias?)
12. Nākinī	Repeated still birth
13. Piśācī	Neonatal death immediate after birth
14. Yakṣī	Neonatal death on 2nd day of birth
15. Āsurī	Neonatal death on 3rd day of birth
16. Kālī	Neonatal death on 4th day

17.	Vāruṇī	Neonatal death on 5th day
18.	Saṣṭhī	Neonatal death on 6th day
19.	Bhīruka	Neonatal death on 7th day
20.	Yāmya	Neonatal death on 8th day
21.	Mātangī	Neonatal death on 9th day
22.	Bhadrakālī	Neonatal death on 10th day
23.	Raudrī	Neonatal death on 11th day
24.	Vardhikā	Neonatal death on 12th day
25.	Candikā	Neonatal death on 13th day
26.	Kapālamalinī	Neonatal death on 14th day
27.	Pilipicchikā	Neonatal death on 15th day
28.	Vaśyā	Intra-uterine death of fetus in 2nd Trimester
29.	Kulakṣa-yakarī	Death of only male children
30.	Puṇyajanī	Death of child immediate after birth
31.	Pauruṣādinī	Death of child before attaining 16 years of life
32.	Sandansī	Death of child after next conception of his mother
33.	Karkoṭakī	Death of one child and affliction by grahas to the other child (out of twins) consequent upon achieving of conception
34.	Indravaḍavā	Death of biovular twins
35.	Baḍavāmukhī	Death of Uniovular twins.

PRINCIPLES OF TREATMENT OF BĀLA-GRAHAS

Suśruta and Vāgbhaṭa both have described the treatment/management of bāla grahas in very detail,[313] however, Vāgbhaṭa has especially mentioned various principles and general measures which play an important role in management of bāla grahas.

The general principles and measures for management of bāla-grahas are as follows:[314]

1. Isolation of child—The seized child be isolated in a separate room, which should be cleaned at least three times in a day. The water should be sprinkled on the ground and fire should be burned continuously in the room. For protection, ash, flowers, seeds, leaves, yava,

tila, sarṣapa, etc. should be scattered in the room and a lamp should be lit with mustard oil.

2. The attendants should follow the rules and should not indulge in various activities like sexual activities and consumption of wine and meat.
3. The affected child should be kept clean by various measures like anointment, bath and fumigation.

(i) Anointment—Old ghṛta (of more than 10 years) is very effective for children affected with grahas.

(ii) Bath—The child should be bathed with lukewarm water, medicated with various drugs like—Balā, Nimba, Agnimantha, Pāribhadra, Śyonāka, Jambū, Vāraṇa, Kaṛtṛṇa, Apāmārga, Paṭola, Śigru (Madhura), Kapittha, Karañja, etc.

These drugs having the properties of astringent, and antiseptic thus may help to keep the child clean and free from various infections. Other measures like isolation of affected child, purification of room and attendants indicate the infectious nature of grahas.

Vāgbhaṭa has mentioned a special type of bath, for child and mother/dhātrī, known as 'Snapana.'

(iii) Fumigation—This procedure is also helpful in keeping the child clean and free from various infections. The following fumigations are effective in all the types of grahas—

(a) Fumigation with the skin of panther, tiger, lion, slough of snake with ghṛta.

(b) Pūtikarañja (its 10 parts like, leaves, root, skin or bark, extract, flowers, fruits, buds, fresh juice, spikes and milk or latex), Bhallātaka, Ajamodā, Kuṣṭha and ghṛta.

(c) Leaves of Sarṣapa and Nimba, root of Aśvakhura, Vacā, Bhūrjapatra with ghṛta.

4. Protection of child by use of Aparājitā—Aprājitā is a special type of therapy, which was used by Buddhists for protection from evil powers.

The Aparājitā after being written by Goracana, should be kept covered along with drugs like Laxamaṇā, Sahadevī, Nāgadantī, Kaṭambharā, Markaṭī, Karkaṭī, Lamba, Bṛhatī, Indrāyaṇa, etc. and should be tied in the neck of the child, after putting all these in Bhūrjapatra. In non-availability of Aparājitā a strong cotton thread should be tied in the neck of child, with enchanting of mantras. This will protect the child from demons.

5. Religious measures—Various religious measures have been also prescribed for relieving the seized child. These include—Japa, bali, and homa.

   (i) Japa—Exchanging of mantras have been considered to allay the bad effects of grahas. For each graha a specific mantra has been described.

   (ii) Bali—The offerings for bali are made according to the likings of the grahas. The following substances should be offered to grahas for getting relief from grahas. These are:

   Flowers—garlands made of red or white flowers.

   Food articles—milk, ghṛta, cooked rice without ghṛta, kṛśarā (khicharī), curd, kulmāṣa, cooked or uncooked meat, fish, wine, etc.

   Drugs—Surasā, Arjaka, Nirguṇḍi (flowers and leaves).

   These above articles should be offered at different places according to graha. The common places for this purpose are—crossings of roads, cemetery, temple, near tree or bell.

   (iii) Homa—The god 'Agni' should be prayed by performing homa (presenting offerings to sacred fire) by 108 times, with various flowers (red coloured), Guggulu, and wooden sticks of Khadira or Candana. Vāgbhaṭa has further described about a specific procedure of homa, known as Agni daṇḍa (power of fire). During performing this procedure the physician should observe the flames of fire which have been said to provide the information, regarding the effect of homa. The child will get cured if the flame becomes red, coppery, like red hot gold; bright like stars, vaidūrya maṇi or moon and exhibits the smell of ghṛta and appearance like red lotus. Opposite to this, if the flame beomes blackish, ash like, or like colour of pigeon and emits odour like fish, blood, pus or garlic; it indicates that the homa is not effective and child may not get relief.

6. Oral use of medicated ghṛtas—Use of following mentioned ghṛtas may prove effective to get rid of various bāla grahas:

   (i) Ghṛta medicated with Anantamūla, Āmrāsthi, Tagara, Marica, Pṛśniparṇī, Mustā, drugs of Madhura gaṇa and decoction of drugs belonging to Daśamūla group.

   (ii) Ghṛta medicated with Rāsnā, Śālaparṇī, Praśniparṇī, Vṛhata pañcamūla, Balā, Mustā, Sārivā, Trikaṭu, Citraka, Pāṭhā, Viḍanga, Madhuyaṣṭhī, Payasyā, Hingu, Devadāru, Granthika and Indrayava.

   (iii) Ghṛta medicated with Sārivā, Surabhi, Brāhmī, Śankhapuṣpī, Kuṣṭha, Saraṣapa, Vacā, Aśvagandhā, Surasā.
   Along with oral use, its massage is also very effective.

   (iv) Ghṛta medicated with Brāhmī, Sarṣapa, Vacā, Sārivā, Kuṣṭha, Pippalī and rock salt is very effective in Graha rogas and known as 'Aṣṭamangala ghṛta'.[315]

Besides these above measures, various specific measures are also described in texts, which should be applied in the management of that specific graha.

L. SOME UNCLASSIFIED SYMPTOMS OR DISORDERS

In ancient texts certain unclassified symptoms or disorders, affecting to the children, are described. Some of these are as follows:

Vicchinna Roga

Vangasena[316] has first time described this disease, but only its treatment. No any description regarding its etiopathogenesis and clinical features are mentioned. However, by the name and type of therapy, it may be considered either the complication of cutting of umbilical cord or any other wound.

Treatment:

(a) Local applications:

(i) Oil medicated with pasted roots of Gorakha-muṇḍī.

(ii) Paste of Āmalakī with cow's urine.

(iii) Pasted seeds of Śālaparṇī and Eraṇḍa.

(b) Massage—Tila oil with powder of Sarja should be used on the affected part.

Parvānuplava

The condition is characterised by pain in different body parts. Initially the pain originate from hand and refered to head, back, muṣka (testicles) and legs. This condition is described by Vāgbhaṭa. Explanation and proper correlation of this disease appear difficult, however, it may be considered as Rheumatoid arthritis.

This painful condition should be treated with massage of oil, medicated with Gaurī (haridrā), Vaca, Arka, Aśvagandhā, Trikaṭu, Kaṭphala, Vārtākī (both types) Āmalakī, Hingu, Rohiṣa, Cow's urine and surā (wine).[317]

REFERENCES

1. C.S.Ci. 30.282-284
2. A.S.U. 2.91
3. A.S.U. 2.92, 93
4. V.S.Bāla. 131
5. A.S.U. 2.92
6. A.H.U. 23.21
7. V.S.Bāla. 129.130
8. A.S.U. 2.85
9. C.S.Śā. 8.44; A.S.U.2.88
10. A.S.U. 2.88; C.D. 64.5; G.N. 11.59
11. C.D. 64.4
12. A.S.U. 2.86
13. A.S.U. 2.87
14. S.S.Śā. 10.34
15. A.S.U. 2.89
16. C.S.Śā. 8.45 Cakara. Comm.
17. A.S.U. 2.90
18. C.D. 64.6
19. C.S.Śā. 8.45
20. C.D. 64.6-17
21. C.S.Ci. 30.232 to 236; S.S.Śā. 8.26, 27; A.S.U. 2.3
22. C.S.Sū. 19.3; C.S.Ci. 30.237
23. S.S.Ni. 10.23
24. A.H.U. 2.4; M.N. 68.4
25. K.S.Sū. 19
26. A.S.U. 2.14-16
27. Hā.S. 3.54.1,2
28. C.S.Śā .8.55; S.S.Ni. 10.23; A.S.U. 2.4,5,6; A.H.U. 2.3,4
29. K.S.Sū.19
30. C.S.Ci. 30.251; S.S.Śā. 10.27; K.S.Sū. 9; A.S.U.1. 38; 2.3,7; A.H.U. 2.1,5; M.N. 67.1, 68.3; K.S.Phakka.; A.S.U. 2.46; A.H.U. 2.44-46.

31. K.S.Sū. 19; A.S.U. 2.14, 16
32. C.S.Sū. 19.13.1; C.S.Ci. 30.237
33. Hā.S. 3.54. 1,2
34. C.S.Śā. 8.56
35. C.S.Ci. 30.251-256
36. S.S.Ci. 17.24, 25,27
37. A.S.U. 2.10; A.H.U.2.9
38. K.S.Sū. 19
39. C.S.Ci. 30.252-253
40. S.S.Ci. 17.24
41. C.S.Ci. 30.254, 255
42. C.S.Sū. 4.18
43. C.S.Śā. 8.56; C.S.Ci. 30.261, 262
44. S.S.Ci. 17.26,27
45. A.S.U. 2.30; A.H.U. 2.34,35
46. A.H.U. 2.25
47. K.S.Sū.19
48. Hā.S. 3.53.2,3
49. A.S.U. 2.11-18; A.H.U. 2.9-26
50. A.SU.2. 12-16
51. C.S.Śā. 8.56; C.S.Ci. 30.257-260; K.S.Sū. 19.
52. C.S.Ci. 30.263-281
53. M.M. Williamm's Sansk. Eng. Dict.
54. C.S.Ci. 28.95
55. A.S.U. 2.46-54
56. K.S.Ci. Phakka.
57. A.S.U. 2.46
58. A.H.U. 2.50
59. A.S.U. 2.54
60. A.S.U. 2.51,53
61. G.N. 11.96-108
62. C.S.Ci. 30.238

63. A.S.U. 2.16
64. C.S.Ci. 30,263,264
65. A.S.U. 2.16
66. A.S.U. 2.60
67. A.H.U. 2.22
68. C.S.Vi. 2.10,11,12
69. A.S.U. 2.60
70. A.S.U. 2.17; A.H.U. 2.20-22; G.N. 11.18.20
71. A.H.U. 2.22
72. C.S.Vi. 2.13
73. A.S.U. 2.18
74. A.H.U. 2.21
75. Y.R.S. Vandhyā. 399-401
76. A.S.U. 2.64
77. A.S.U. 2.64; M.N. 68.11; G.N. 11.127, 128
78. A.S.U. 2.64; V.S.70.102
79. A.S.U. 2.66; G.N.11.129-131
80. A.S.U. 2.71
81. K.S.Ci. Phakka.
82. K.S.Ci. Phakka.
83. A.S.U. 2.74
84. M.N. 68.12, 13; G.N. 11.132, 133; V.S. Bāla. 103, 104
85. V.V. 69.8.
86. S.S.Śā. 10.47; A.S.U. 2.75-78; G.N. 11.134, 135; V.S. Bāla. 106
87. S.S.Śā. 10.47
88. C.D. 47; G.N. 11.72; V.S. 105-109, 113
89. C. Kalikā. Kaumā. 379; V.S. Bāla. 107-109
90. C.S.Ci. 19.3; S.S.U. 40.5
91. C. Kalikā. Kaumā. 378; H.M. 4.346; C.D. 64.31; G.N.Ci. 11.45; V.S. 70.32; A.S.U. 2.42
92. C.D. 64.35
93. C.D. 64.32

94. V.S. 70.36, 37
95. V.S. 70.39
96. G.N.Ci. 11.119
97. A.S.U. 2.35
98. V.S. 70.46
99. V.S. 70.47
100. V.S. 70.43
101. Hā.S. 3.54.19
102. A.S.U. 2.35
103. V.S. 70.42; V.V.(9) 7
104. V.S. 70.45
105. A.S.U. 2.35
106. Y.R.S. Vandhyā. 448, 449, 454
107. C.D. 64.38
108. G.N. 11.64
109. Hā. S.3.3
110. S.S.Vi. 40
111. C.S.Ci. 15
112. C.D. 64.42
113. C.D. 64.43
114. V.S. 70.161, 162
115. S.S.U. 49
116. Harmekh. 4.347
117. C.D. 64.29; V.S. 70.71, 173
118. A.H.U. 2.59
119. V.S. 7.74
120. V.S. 70.67
121. A.S.U. 2.57
122. A.S.U. 2.57; G.N. 11.63
123. A.S.U. 2.58
124. S.S.U. 48
125. A.S.U. 2.58

126. A.S.U. 2.36
127. Y.R.S. Vandhyā. 465
128. C.D. 64.58
129. R.M. Bāla.
130. C.D. Bāla.59
131. V.S. 70.51, 52
132. S.S. Śā. 10.49; Cikitsā K. 379; V.V. 69. 15; C.D. 66.44; G.N. 11.69
133. Hā.S. 3.54.9-13
134. C.S.Ci. 18.6-8
135. C.S.Ci. 18; S.S.U. 52
136. A.S.U. 2.55
137. A.H.U. 2.57; Y.R.S. Vandhyā. 456; C.K. Kumār. 380 V.V. 69.11
138. V.V. 69.22; G.N. 11.68
139. V.S. 70.58
140. V.S. 70.59
141. V.S. 70.69
142. Hā.S. 54.16
143. S.S.U. 51
144. C.S.Ci. 17.17
145. A.S.U. 2.56; V.S. 70.45
146. C.D. 64.55
147. Y.R.S. Vandhyā. 554
148. V.V. 69.21; C.D. 64.56; G.N. 11.67
149. V.S. 70.60
150. K.S.Khil. Chapt.13
151. C.D. 64.60
152. G.N.Ci. 11.126
153. C.D. 64.61
154. Hā.S. 54.21
155. S.S.U. 19.9,10; K.S. Khil. 3; M.N. Bāla. 9
156. A.S.U. 2.19.

157. S.S.Sū. 19.9
158. K.S.Khil. 3.5
159. S.S.U. 19.9, 10; K.S. Khil. 9.11; A.H.U. 8.19,20
160. K.S.Khil. 13
161. A.S.U. 9.24,25
162. K.S.Khil. 13
163. A.H.U. 2.79
164. S.S.Ni. 13.59; A.S.U. 2.79; A.H.U. 2.69
165. S.S.Ni. 13.60; A.S.U. 2.79; A.H.U. 2.70
166. S.S.Ci. 20.57; A.S.U. 2.80
167. S.S.Ci. 20.58; A.S.U. 2.80
168. S.S.Ci. 20.59
169. A.S.U. 2.80; A.H.U. 2.73; G.N.Ci. 11.141
170. A.S.U. 2.80
171. A.H.U. 2.74
172. V.S. 70.112
173. S.S.Ci. 20.59
174. A.S.U. 2.80
175. A.S.U. 2.81
176. S.S.Ci. 20.57
177. A.S.U. 2.80; V.S. 70.112
178. K.S.Khil. 15
179. C.S.Ci. 7.24; S.S.Ni. 5
180. K.S.Khil. 15.6
181. K.S.Khil. 15.7
182. K.S.Khil. 15.4,5
183. C.S.Ci. 7.24
184. S.S.Ni. 5.10
185. K.S.Khil. 15.4
186. K.S.Khil. 15.6
187. K.S.Khil. 15.7-10
188. K.S.Khil. 15.11

189. K.S. Khil. 15.12.14
190. K.S. Khil. 15.15.17
191. K.S.Khil. 14.4.5
192. C.S.Ci. 21.11
193. K.S.Khil. 14.9; S.S.Ni. 5.5
194. C.S.Ci. 21.15
195. C.S.Ci. 21. 17-21
196. K.S.Khil. 14.10.14
197. A.H.N. 13.47-65; K.S.Khil. 14.15; C.S. 21.12-14
198. S.S.Ni. 10.4-7
199. K.S.Khil. 14
200. C.S.Ci. 21.115
201. A.S.U. 2.61
202. V.S.Bāla. 79-83
203. V.S.Bāla. 114-119
204. S.S.Su. 27.10; A.S.Su. 3.15
205. A.S.U. 2.94
206. S.S.Ni. 13.4
207. S.S.Ci. 20.3-4
208. K.S.Ci. Dvivṛṇīya.
209. K.S.Ci. Dvivṛṇīya.
210. K.S.Ci. Dvivṛṇīya.
211. M.N. 54.13
212. S.S.Ci. 1.6
213. S.S.Ci. 1.3; K.S.Ci. Dvivṛṇā. 7
214. K.S.Ci. Dvivṛṇā.
215. K.S.Ci. Dvivṛṇā. 10.25
216. C.S.Su. 17.82, 83; S.S.Ni. 6.16
217. K.S.Ci. Dvivṛṇā.
218. S.S.Ni. 3.3.,11
219. S.S.Ni. 3.4.,11
220. S.S.Ni. 3.3,25

221. S.S.Ni. 3.5,6
222. S.S.Ni. 3.8-10; K.S.Sū. Vedanā. 25.24; A.S.U. 2.9
223. S.S.Ni. 3.8-10; C.S.Ci. 26.37
224. S.S.Ci. 7.3
225. S.S.Ci. 7.4
226. S.S.Ci. 7.30-34
227. K.S.Ci. Mūtra.
228. S.S.U. 59.3
229. C.S.Ci. 26.34, 35
230. C.S.U. 59.3; K.S.Ci. Mūtra.
231. K.S.Ci. Mūtra.
232. M.N. 31.1
233. Y.R.S. Vandhyā. 469; V.V. 69.16; C.D.Bāla. 64.45; G.N. 11.70
234. V.S.Bāla. 126-128
235. C.S.Ci. 3.26
236. S.S.U. 39.13
237. C.S.Ni. 1.17; C.S.Ci. 3.90
238. C.S.Ni. 1.19
239. C.S.Ni. 1.36
240. K.S.Khil. 2.3
241. Y.R.S.Vandhyā.
242. C.S.Ci. 16.3
243. C.S.Ci. 16.7-11
244. C.S.Ci. 16.12
245. C.S.Ci. 16.34-36
246. A.V. 2.32.1; 4.20.9; 2.31.2; 8.3.15; 8.6.9; 2.31.4; R.V. 10.162
247. C.S.Ci. 16.36
248. C.S.Ci. 16.39-43
249. C.S.Ci. 16.118-123
250. A.S.U. 2.95
251. A.S.U. 2.38-40'; G.N. 11.65,66
252. A.V.V. 23.2
253. C.S.Sū. 19.9; S.S.U. 54.7; A.S.Ni. 14

254. A.S.Ni. 14.43-45
255. M.N. 7.4; S.S.V. 54.18, 19
256. A.V. 2.32.1
257. C.S.Vi. 7.14,15
258. K.S.Ci. Kṛimi.
259. C.S.Vi. 7.16
260. K.S.Ci. Kṛimi.
261. Pāṇinī.III. 3.58
262. M.Bh.Vana. 230.43
263. A.V.III. 2.1
264. K.S. 26.14, 21, 26-32
265. A.V.II. 2.25.3; R.V.10.162
266. K.S.20.1-3
267. P.G.S. 1.16.24; A.G.S. 2.7; B.G.S. 3.7.27
268. M.Bh.Vana. 230, Ādiparva. 66.24, Śalya. 43.37, Sabhā. 11.41
269. M.Bh.Vāna. 229.1-3, 230.24-30,; Śalya. 46.15, 18, 21, 24, 26, 34, 35
270. Mārkaṇdeya Pu.
271. C.S.Sū .6.27
272. S.S.U. 27.4.20
273. A.S.U. 3.2
274. K.S.Sū. 19
275. K.S.Indriya. 5.1.13-21
276. K.S. Ci.Bālagraha
277. K.S.Kalpa. Revatī.
278. A.V.II. 2.25.3; R.V. 10.162
279. K.K. 18
280. C.D.Bāla. 84-107; Hā.S.
281. K.S.Revatī.Kalpā.
282. S.S.U. 60.19
283. S.S.U. 27.6; S.S.U. 37.18-20
284. A.H.U. 3.32
285. S.S.Śā. 10.51; A.H.U. 3.4, 5

286. S.S.U. 37.8, 28
287. S.S.U. 27.8
288. A.S.U 3.5-8
289. S.S.U. 37.7; S.S.U. 29.9
290. S.S.U. 27.9; A.S.U. 3.11
291. S.S.U. 36.1, 2, 11
292. S.S.U. 27.16; A.S.U. 3.12
293. S.S.U. 32.12
294. S.S.U. 27.12; A.S.U. 3.16
295. S.S.U. 34.9
296. S.S.U. 27.14; A.S.U. 3.17
297. S.S.U. 33.10
298. S.S.U. 27.13; A.S.U. 3.18
299. A.S.U. 6.29
300. A.S.U. 3.14
301. A.S.U. 6.23
302. A.S.U. 3.13
303. S.S.U. 31.10
304. S.S.U. 27.11; A.S.U. 3.20
305. A.S.U. 3.21; 6.54
306. A.S.U. 3.21; 6.54
307. S.S.U. 30.12, 13
308. S.S.U. 27.10; A.S. U.3.15
309. S.S.U. 35.10
310. S.S.U. 27.15; A.S.U. 3.19
311. Agni Purāṇa Bāla. 2.99
312. K.S.Kalpa. Revatī.
313. S.S.U. 28-37; A.S.U. 4.6
314. A.S.U. 4,5
315. V.S. 70.176, 178; G.N. 11.87-89; C.D. 64.74-76
316. V.S. 70.20-24
317. A.S.U. 2.73

Bibliography

A Sanskṛit - English Dictionary; Sir Monier Monior Williams; Motilal Banarsidas, Delhi (1984).

A Critical Appraisal of Āyurvedic Material in Buddhist Literature with Special Reference to Tripitak; Dr. Jyotir Mitra; Published by Jyotiralok Prakashan, Varanasi (1985).

A Short History of Aryan Medical Science; Bhagvat Singh; New Asian Publishers, Delhi (1978).

Abhinava Bāla Tantra; Jain, C.M. and Sharma, V.P.; Chaukhamba Surbharati Prakasana, Varanasi (1990).

Alberuni's India; Edward, C. Sachaw, Vol.I, II; S. Chand & Co., Delhi (1964).

APGAR, V., A Propoal for New Method of Evaluation of the Newborn Infant Anesth. Analg. 32: 260 (1953).

Atharva Veda (Śaunakīya) with Sayana Commentary, Part I & IV, edited by Vishwa Bandhu; Vishveshwaranand Vedic Research Institute, Hoshiarpur (1961).

Agni Purāṇa Kī Darshanika Evam Āyurvedic Samagrī Kā Adhyayana; Dr. Sarita Handa; Jyotiralok Prakashan, Varanasi (1982).

Antiquities of India; L.D. Burnett, Punthi Pustaka, Calcutta (1964).

Aṣṭānga Saṃgraha 'Sarwānga-Sundary' Commentary; edited by Pt. Lalchandra Sharma; Vaidyanath Ayurveda Bhawan Pvt. Ltd., Patna.

Aṣṭānga Hṛdaya of Vāgbhaṭa with Vidyotinī Commentary by Kaviraj Atrideva Gupta, edited by Yadunandan Upadhyaya, Chowkhamba Sanskrit Sansthan, Varanasi (1975).

Āyurvediya Prasūti Tantra Evam Strī Roga, Part I; Dr. (Km.) Premvati Tewari; Chaukhamba Orientalia; Varanasi (1986).

Āyurvedīya Pañcakarma-Vijjanna (Hindi), Vaidya Haridas Shridhar Kasture Published by Sri Vaidyanath Ayurveda Bhawan Ltd., Nagpur (1985).

Bāla-Veda, Edited and Published for Pediatric Clinics of India by V.B. Athavale, 206, Sion Road, Bombay (1977).

Bṛhata Jātaka of Varāhamihira by V. Subramanya Sastri, First Ed., Govt. Branch Press, Mysore (1929).

Breast Feeding in Practice; Elisabet Helsing; Oxford University Press, Delhi (1984).

Caraka Saṃhitā with 'Ayurveda Deepika' Commentary by Cakrapanidutta; Edited by Yadava ji Trikramji Acharya, Chowkhamba Sanskrit Sansthan, Varanasi (1984).

Cakradatta of Sri Cakrapāṇidatt with the 'Bhāvārth Sandīpinī, Hindi Commentary by J.P. Tripathi, Chowkhamba Sanskrit Series Office, Varanasi (1983).

Cikitsā Kalikā by Tīsaṭāchrya with the Commentary of Candrata, Edited by Kaviraj Narendra Nath Mitra and Translated by Jayadeva, Pub. by Mitra Ayurvedic Pharmacy, Lahore (1926).

Clinical Embryology; Richard S. Smell; Asian Edition; Little, Brown and Company, Boston (1983).

Common Symptoms of Diseases in Children, R.S. Illingworth; Oxford University Press, N. Delhi (1989).

Divyāvadāna; Ed. P.L. Vaidya, Mithila Vidyapith, Darbhanga, Bihar (1958).

Essentials of Human Embryology; A.K. Datta; Current Book International, Bombay (1978).

Ekādaśopaniṣad; Published by Motilal Banarsi Das, Delhi (1966).

Functional Human Anatomy; 2nd Edition; James E. Crouch; Lea & Feriger, Philadelphia (1972).

Elliot, G.B. and Ellot, K.A., Some Pathological, Radiological and Clinical Implications of the Precarious Development of the Human Ear; Laryngoscope 74; 1160-1171 (1964).

Findlay, A.L.R.; Res. Reprod. 6, 6 Neural and Behavioural Interaction with Lactation, Butterworth, London (1974).

Gobhilagṛhyasūtram; Edited by Chintamani Bhattacharya, Published by Munshiram Manoharlal Publishers Pvt. Ltd. (1982).

Gray's Anatomy; Edited by Carmine D. Clemente; 13th American Edition, K.M. Varghese Company, P.B. 7119, Bombay (1985).

Harṣa Carita; Commentator—Mohan Deva Pant, Motilal Banarasidas, Delhi (1984).

Harṣa Charitam of Banabhatta; Edited with the 'Sanketa Sanskrit Comm. of Sankara Kavi & Hindi Translation by Pt. Jagannath Pathak; Chowkhambha Vidya Bhawan, Varanasi (1982).

Harmekhalā of Mahuka Part I & II; Edited by K. Sambasiva Sastri, Printed by Government Press, Trivandum (1936).

Hārīta Saṃhitā; Published by Khemraj Shrikrishnadas, Sri Venkateswar Press (1927).

Hearing in Children; Jerry L. Northern Marion P. Downs; IInd. Ed., The Williams and Wilkins Co., Baltimore, Maryland, USA (1978).

Hindu Saṃskāra by Dr. Rajbali Panday, Chowkhamba Vidyabhawan, Varanasi (1978).

History of Dharma Śāstra (Part I to V) by Dr. P.V. Kane; Published by Govt. of U.P., Rajarshi Purushottam Das Hindi Bhawan, Lucknow.

History of Civilization in Ancient India (Based on Sanskrit Literature), Vol. I & II by R.C. Dutta; Vishal Publishers, Delhi-6 (1972).

Human milk in the modern world; Derrick B. Jelliffe; E.F. Patrice Jelliffe; Oxford University Press, Oxford, New York (1978).

Human Nutrition and Dietetics; Sir Stanley Davidson; R. Passmore, J.F. Brocle; A.S. Truswell; 6th Ed., The ELBS & Churchill Livingstone, Edinburgh (1975).

Human Embroylogy; Inderbir Singh; MacMillan India Limited, Delhi (1982).

Hytten (1954); Clinical and Chemical Studies in Human Lactation; VII Relationship of the Age, Physique and Nutritional Status of the Mother to the Yield and Composition of Her Milk; Br. Med. Jr. (i), 844-5.

Jaiminīya Brāhmaṇa; Edited by Raghu Vira; International Academy of Indian Culture, Nagpur (1954).

Kaumārbhṛtyantargata bālagrahon Kā Kramika Evam Vaijnanik Adhyayan; Ph.D. Thesis of Dr. C.K. Sharma, Kameshwar Singh Darbhanga Sanskrit University, Darbhanga (1985).

Kalyāṇakāraka by Ugardityacharya; Pub. by Seth Govinda Ji Rav ji Doshi, Solapur (1940).

Kauṭilya Arthaśāṣtra; Edited by Dr. Raghu Nath Singh Krishnadas Academy, Varanasi (1983).

Kaśyapa Saṃhitā (Vṛddha Jivakiya Tantra) by Vrddha Jivaka, with The Vidyotini Hindi Commentary, The Chaukhambha Sanskrit Sansthan, Varanasi (1939).

Kādambarī of Bāṇabhaṭṭa, Edited by Sri K.M. Shastri, The Chowkhamba Sanskrit Series Office, Varanasi (1961).

Kālidāsa's Vision of Kumārasambhava; Suryakant; Mehar Chand Lakshman Das, Delhi (1963).

Kumārasambhava of Kālıdasa; Edited by Pradyumna Pandey, Chowkhamba Vidyabhawan, Varanasi (1981).

Longman's Medical Embryology; T.W. Sadler; Williams & Wilkins, Baltimore (USA) (1985).

Lalitvistāra, Published by Mithila Vidyapith, Darbhanga, Bihar (1967).

Levin, B. Mackay, et al. (1959); Weight Gains, Serum Protein Levels and Health of Breast-fed and Artificially-fed Infants. MRC Special Report Series, No. 296, London.

Lipton E.L.; Steinschneider, A. and Richamand, J. (1966) : Auditory Sensitivity in the Infant; Effect of

Intensity on Cardiac and Motor Responsivity; Child Dev. 37:233.

Manu Smṛti Commentory Pt. Keshava Prasad Sharma, Pub. by Khan Raj Srikrishadas, Sri Venkateswar Press, Bombay (1961).

Mahābhārata, Edited by Vishnu S. Sukhankar, Bhandarkar Oriental Research Institute, Poona (1948).

Mahāyān Granthon Mein Nihita Ayurvedic Samagri Ka Adhyayan; Ph.D. Thesis, R.N. Tripathi, AIHC & A. Department, BHU, Varanasi (1983).

Mārkaṇḍeya Purāṇa; Edited by F. Eden Pargiter, Indological Book House, Delhi, Pub. by The Asiatic Society of Bengal (1969).

Mādhava Nidāna of Sri Madhuvakara with Vidyotini Commentary by Shri Sudarsana Sastri, Part II; Chowkhambha Sanskrit Sansthan, Varanasi, (2041).

Mrichchakaṭikam of Sudraka; Edited with 'Bhava Prakashika' Sanskrit-Hindi Comm., by Dr. J.S.L. Tripathi; Krishna Das Academy, Varanasi (1986).

McCarthy, P.H., Delan, T.F.; Hyperpyrexia in Children; A.M.J. Dis. Child. 1976. 13 : 849.

Mother and Child Welfare (Kaumarbhrtyam); A.L. Pathi, V.S. Rao; Devanagri Power Press, Guntur (1955).

Mūlasarvastivāda Vinaya Vastu, Part I, II S.S. Baghchi, Published by Mithila Vidyapith, Darbhanga, Bihar (1967).

Nelson Textbook of Pediatrics; Victor, C. Vaughan, R. James McKay, Richard E. Behrman; W.B. Saunders Company, Philadelphia (1979).

Outlines of the History of Medicine; by Joh. Hermann Baas, Robert E. Krieger; Publishing Co. Inc. Huntington, New York (1971).

Patten's Human Embryology; Clark Edward Corliss; McGraw-Hill Book Company, New York (1976).

Principles and Practice of Paediatrics in Ayurveda: Dr. C.N.S. Shastry, Ph.D. Thesis, Banaras Hindu University (1976).

Pañchakarma-Therapy in Āyurveda by D. Ojha and Ashok Kumar, Chaukhamba Amarkabharati Prakashan, Varanasi (1978).

Pañchakarma Treatment of Ayurveda by Dr. T.L. Devaraj, Dhanwantari Oriental Publications (1980).

Pāraskar Grihya Sūtra; Edited by Mahadeva Gangadhar Bakre; Pub. Munshiram Manoharlal Publishers Pvt. Ltd. (1982).

Ṛg Veda Saṃhitā Commentary by Sayanacarya; Edited by F. Max Muller, Vol. I to IV; Krishnadas Academy, Varanasi (1983).

Śatapatha Brāhmaṇa; Edited by Pt. A. Chinnaswami Shastri; Chowkhamba Sanskrit Sansthan, Varanasi (1984).

Sharma, P.V.; Indian Medicine in the Classical Age; Chowkhamba Publications.

Sāmavidhāna Brāhmaṇa; Critically Edited by Dr. B.R. Sharma, Kendriya Sanskrit Vidyapeeth, Tirupati (1964).

Sacred Books of the East; Edited by F. Max Muller; Vol. XII, XXVI, XLIV, XXX, XXIX, Motilal Banarsi Das, Delhi (1969).

Schaffer's Diseases of the Newborn; Marg Ellen Avery, H. William Taeusch; W.B. Saunders Company, USA, 5th Ed. (1984).

Suśruta Saṃhitā with 'Āyurvedatatva Sandīpikā' Commentary Part I by Dr. A.D. Shastri; The Chowkhamba Sanskrit Sansthan, Varanasi (1972).

Suśruta Saṃhitā (Uttartantram); Commentator Kvj. Dr. Ambika Dutta Shastri, Chowkhamba Sanskrit Series Office, Varanasi (1974).

Status of Kaumārabhṛtya in Ancient India; Dr. Abhimanyu Kumar; Thesis for Doctor of Philosophy, Institute of Medical Sciences, B.H.U. Varanasi (1990).

The Cult of Skanda-Kartikeya in Ancient India; Chatterjee, K.A.; Pub. by Punthi Pustaka, Calcutta (1970).

The Grihya-Sutrass, Edited by Max Muller, Translated by Hermann Oldenberg, Part I & II, Motilal Banarasidas, Varanasi (1964).

The Hindu Medicine (3000 BC to 1200 AD) by A.K. Mazumdar; City Publishing House, Faridabad (Dacca) (1920).

The Developing Human; Keith L. Moore; W.B. Saunders Company, London (1974).

The Wonder that was India; Basham, A.L.; Pub. Sidgwick and Jackson, London (1961).

Taxila, An Illustrasted Account of Archaeological Excavations; by Sir John Marshall; Vol. I, II, III; Motial Banarasi Das, Delhi (1975).

Textbook of Paediatric Nutrition; Edited by Donald S. McLaren and David Burman, 2nd Ed.; Churchill Livingstone, Edinburgh (1982).

Textbook of Human Embroylogy; R. Padmanbhan; CBS Publishers and Distributors, Delhi (1984).

Textbook of Anatomy; W. Henry Holinshead, Cornelius Rose; Harper & Row, Publishers, Philadelphia (1985).

Vakil, Rustam, Jal; Our Glorious Heritage; Times of India Press (1965).

Vaidika Sāhitya Kā Itihās; Paras Nath Dwivedi; Chowkhamba Sanskrit Prakashana, Varanasi (1983).

Vedon Me Āyurveda; Rama Gopal Shastri; Madan Mohan Ayurvedic Research Trust, Delhi (1956).

Viṣṇusmṛti; Edited by Pandit V. Krishnamacharya, Part I & II, Published by the Adyar Library and Research Centre, Madras.

Vṛnda Vaidyaka; Pub. by Khemraj Srikrishnadas & Sri Venkateswar Press, Bombay (1904).

Warkany J., Kalter H. (1961); Congenital Malformations; N. Engl. J. Med. 265; 993.

Yajur Veda, Sāyaṇa Commentary; Edited by Sriram Sharma, Sanskriti Sansthan, Bareilly (1962).

Yājnavalkya Smṛti of Yogishwara Yajnavalkya with Mitaksara Commentary of Vijnaneshwar; Edited by Dr. Umesh Chandra Panday, The Chowkhamba Sanskrit Series Office, Varanasi (1967).

Index